DUMBBELL TRAINING: FOR MEN AND WOMEN

BY

PAUL NAM

OTHER BOOKS BY THE AUTHOR

FIT TO FAT IN 8 WEEKS

SCRAWNY TO BRAWNY IN 8 WEEKS

NUTRITION 101: BUILDING THE FOUNDATION

IMMUNE SYSTEM 8: BOOST YOUR IMMUNE SYSTEM NATURALLY

IT'S ALL ABOUT YOUR HEALTH: FOOD RECIPES

THE BOOK OF CHOICES: THE LIVES OF 2 ATHLETES

BODYBUILDING AND STEROIDS: MY PERSONAL STORY

THE ULTIMATE GUIDE TO CORE(ABS) TRAINING: NO MORE LOW BACK PAIN

DUMBBELL AND CORE(ABS) TRAINING COMBINED

LEARN HOW TO STRETCH FOR BETTER MOVEMENT AND HEALTH

BEGINNER'S GUIDE TO DIET AND TRAINING

TABLE OF CONTENTS

INTRODUCTION

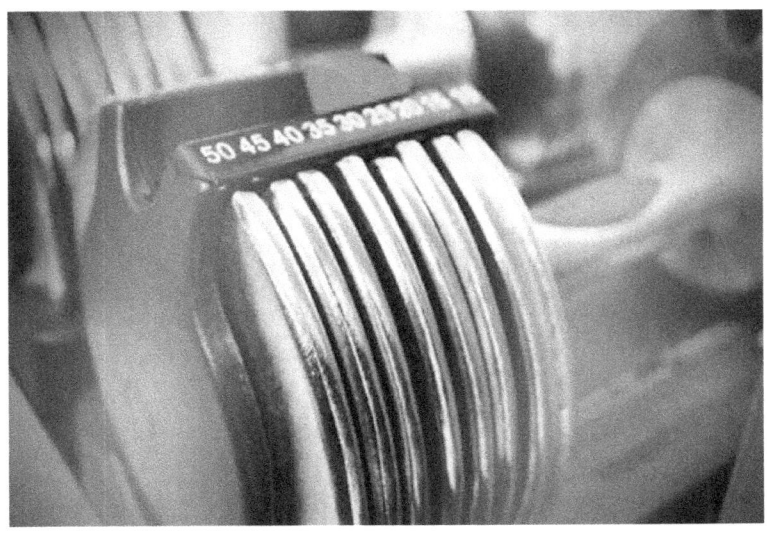

Dumbbells were created in the early 1900's to sculpt the human physique to perfection. Dumbbells are a form of resistance training and they assist to build the skeletal muscle mass in the human body. A few known benefits are tendon strengthening and increased mobility. Did you know increasing your muscle mass helps to increase your basal metabolic rate which burns more calories at rest? As we age our muscle mass decreases so it is important to include some form of training in your everyday life.

Welcome to Dumbbell Training: For Men and Women. This book was created so you can workout at home or use these exercises and incorporate them into your training routine. So get those dumbbells out and get ready to burn some calories!

WHY USE DUMBBELLS?

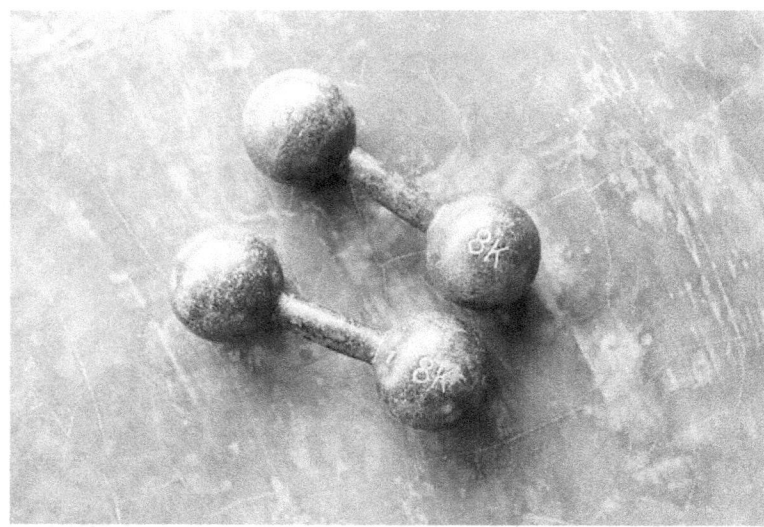

Signing up for a gym membership sounds like a good idea until you get there. When you get to the weight room, you look around in awe. All you see is different types of machines that could be used to torture someone. A rather large freaky looking human being is lifting tremendous amounts of weights on his back. His veins are popping out and it looks like he is going to give birth to a child. Okay, let's get back to the chapter before I start writing about another story. Here is the question most people wonder about. Should I use free weights or machines?

There are benefits and drawbacks to both machines and free weights, and some exercises tend to be more effective when using one or the other.
Hand weights are inexpensive, portable, and readily available for purchase in just about any department store. Keeping them in your living room or office will allow you to exercise whenever you have the time.

The benefit of a resistance machine is that it will allow you to focus your mind on the effort, as opposed to the mechanics of the movement. But, unless you have enough space for a machine in your home, you'll need a gym membership.

The primary difference between free weights and machines, however, is the fact that when using free weights, you can move your body in three dimensions: forward, backward, horizontally, and vertically. This is important, because this is how your body normally moves in daily life.

When you use free weights, you therefore end up using more muscles, as you have to work to stabilize the weight while lifting it. The only drawback is that you're at an increased risk of injury unless you maintain proper form. Always use a lighter weight to get the proper form first before graduating to a heavier weight.

Machines are fixed to an axis that will only allow you to move in one or two planes. If machine are only used, this could lead to a lack of functional fitness, which may lead into injuries outside the gym.

For functional fitness, dumbbells and free weights are far superior than machines. I use both machines and free weights in my routine. If I had a choice to do a dumbbell bench press or a machine bench press, I would chose the dumbbells. The dumbbells give me a greater range of motion which results in greater muscle recruitment.

BENEFITS OF STRENGTH TRAINING

Strength training benefits your:

- Body composition – positive change in your fat to lean body mass ratio
- Blood glucose control – helps to lower blood glucose levels
- Blood pressure – helps to lower blood pressure
- Bone Density – helps to increase bone density mass
- Cardiorespiratory fitness and aerobic capacity – makes your heart stronger so it has to work less at rest

MUSCLE SUMMARIES

Knowing what exercises work what body part is important for building the mind to muscle connection. When you build the mind to muscle connection, you achieve greater muscle recruitment which results in a greater workout.

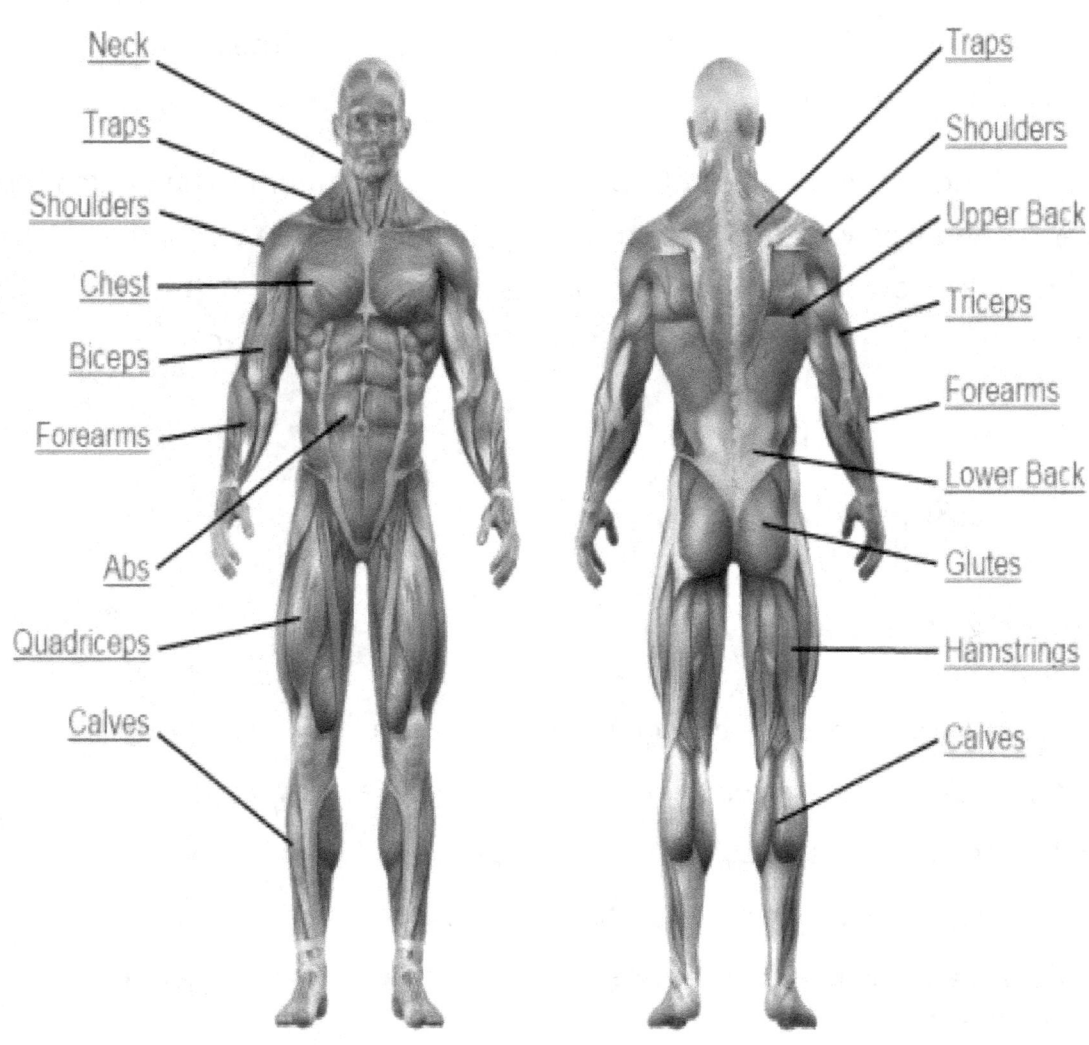

Chest

The chest muscle is composed of the pectoralis major and pectoralis minor. Exercises such as the bench press and push-ups are good exercises that target this muscle. Chest muscles help to push things like a grocery cart and assist with actions like closing a door.

Abdominal(Abs)

The abdomen makes up the area between the chest and pelvis. Exercises like crunches work the upper abs while exercises like scissor kicks work the lower abs. They provide a key role in providing posture and stability for the body during movement. They also act as protection for the stomach. You use your ab muscles every time you get out of bed and lie down.

Serratus

The serratus muscle originates from the upper ribs and extends to the spinal area. Exercises like dumbbell pullovers work the serratus. This muscle allows us to move our arms around multi/-dimensionally. They are responsible for providing support and balance in the arms and shoulders. They are used in activities like turning a wheel when you drive.

Obliques

The oblique muscles occupy the outer abdomen area. One exercise that works this particular area is the dumbbell side tilt. They help to support the rotation of the spine and help to bend the torso. When you bend sideways to pick up your pencil this muscle gets worked.

Middle/Outer Back

Middle and outer back muscles are composed of latissumis dorsi, rhomboids, teres major, and teres minor. Exercises that mostly work the lats are pull downs and chin ups. Barbell back rows and all rowing movements work the rhomboids, teres major, and teres minor. The back supports everyday posture and helps with movements like opening a door.

Lower Back

The low back muscles covers the lumbar spine. Exercises that work this area are bird dogs and land swimming. Exercises are important to keep this area strong. The low back is one of the most common areas of the body that is strained. Every time you bend over and shovel snow you activate this muscle.

Trapezius

A pair of large triangular muscles that cover most of the upper back including the posterior part of the neck. Dumbbell or barbell shrugs target this muscle effectively. One of the major functions of the trap muscles is to support the weight carried by the arms. Basically when you lift or carry anything you activate these muscles.

Deltoids

The delt muscle is formed around the edges of the shoulder and ends at the middle of the arm. This muscle is made up of the anterior, medial, and posterior head. Barbell or machine front presses work this muscle. When you reach upwards to grab those dishes you work these muscles.

Biceps

The biceps attaches from the shoulder and ends at the forearm. The long head and short head make up this muscle. Dumbbell or barbell curls work the biceps. You work this muscle when you carry your bag of groceries.

Triceps

The triceps muscle makes up about 2/3rd of the arm. They are composed of the medial, long, and short head. Exercises that work the triceps are cable push downs and dumbbell overhead extensions. Pushing your grocery cart down the isle works this muscle.

Glutes

Gluteus medius and maximus make up this muscle. They are located between the pelvis and the hamstrings. Glute maximus is one of the strongest muscles in the body and is responsible for the movement of the hips and thighs. Compound exercises like the squats and lunges work the glute muscles.

Quadriceps

The quads are composed of 4 muscles. The vastus medialis, vastus lateralis, rectus femoris, vastus intermedius. They are located on the front part of the leg and allow movement for the knee. Your quads are one of the largest body parts so training them burns more calories. Squats, lunges, and leg presses are good exercises for this muscle. Getting up from a chair works these muscles.

Hamstrings

The hamstrings are made up of the semitendinosus, semibranosus, and biceps femoris. They span from the gluteal muscles to the knee. Stiff legged dead lifts works this muscle. When you ride a bike you activate this muscle.

Calves

The calf muscle is composed of the soleus and gastrocenemius which is located on the back of the lower leg. Seated and standing calf raises work these muscles. Basic activities like walking and running work these muscles. Since we use calves for movement it is important to keep them strong and flexible.

TRAINING GUIDELINES

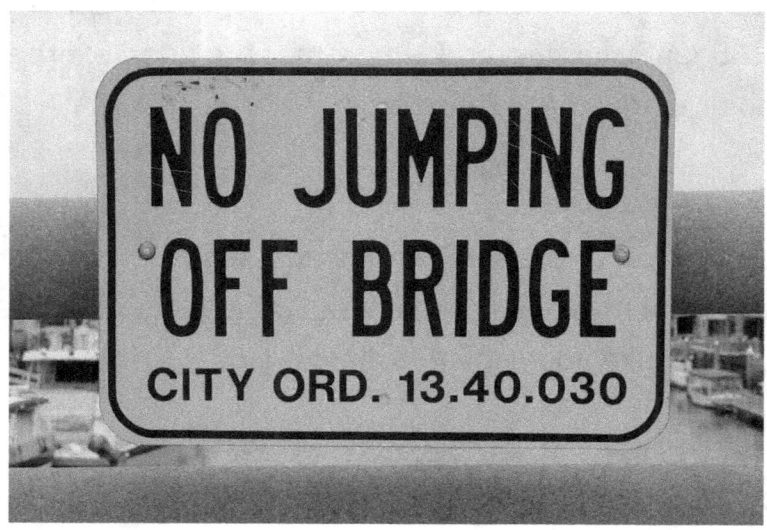

1. Always use good form. A good controlled set will recruit more muscle fibres verses throwing the weight around.

2. Do 1 set with a lighter weight. Then increase the weight for the next set and then increase the weight for the next set. If you can complete 10-12 with proper form then increase the weight by 5-10 lbs.

3. Lower the weight in a controlled motion. To many people forget about the negative portion (lowering) as this is just as important as the lifting.

4. Breath out with force. Never hold your breath while during exercise or a set. Your muscles need oxygen to keep working and being red in the face doesn't look to good.

5. Know when to stop and when to push yourself. Training with out any rest days and pushing yourself too hard can result in an injury or over training.

6. Record your weights in a book so you know what you did before. This is a way to progress.

7. Do large muscle groups before smaller muscle groups. Doing triceps before chest is suicide. Your triceps will fatigue before your chest.

8. Set goals and work towards them. This will help you focus more.

10. Never train right after a meal. Best to wait at least 1.5 to 2 hours after solid food. Your digestive tract needs the energy to digest your food so if you train your food will sit undigested in your stomach.

11. Always do a 5-8 minute warm up. If you start lifting weights right away you risk yourself for an injury and this does not give your body a proper start to training.

12. Always lift in a controlled manner and do not do speed reps unless you are training for something specific. Explosive movements are dangerous unless done under supervision of a certified trainer.

13. Always do a 5-8 minutes cool down. As your body needs to warm up it needs to cool down also. This gives it time to bring your heart rate back to a normal range.

14. An example of a warm up and a cool down is a fast paced walk on a treadmill or outside.

15. Use a steady tempo when lifting weights. A tempo like 3-0-3-0 usually works well. This means 3 seconds upwards, no rest at top, 3 seconds downwards, and no rest at the bottom.

16. Always include some form of stretching after. It is best to do static stretching after your training. If you need some ideas on stretching, download my Stretch Fitness app for Android. Just follow the website link (www.pursefitness.com) and click on the Android button. It will take you to all the Android apps.

17. If you need some ideas on core(abs) training, download my Core Fitness app for Android.

NUTRITIONAL GUIDELINES

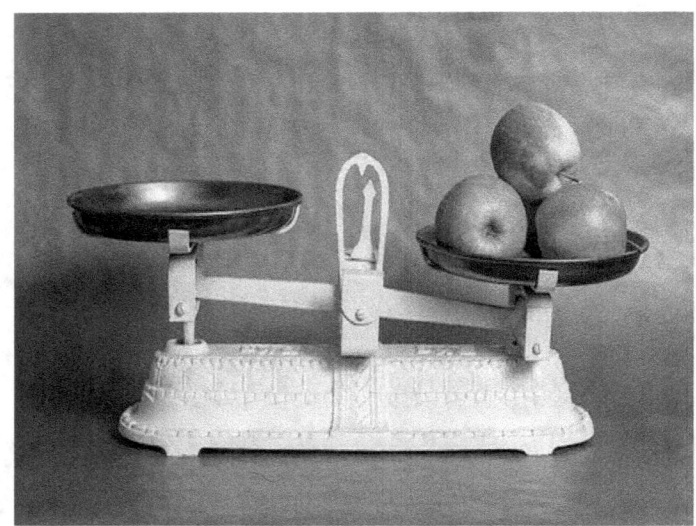

If your goal is fat loss then follow these guidelines.

Men

1. Figure out your basal metabolic rate (BMR) and make sure it matches your caloric intake. If you are eating under your BMR and feel full, do not add extra calories in. For faster fat loss stay 200-300 calories below your BMR.

2. Drink 8-12 glasses of water a day.

3. Eat or have a snack every 2.5-3 hours. This maintains homeostasis in your body.

4. Snacks can by nuts, chia seeds, protein shakes, protein bars, cheese, beef jerky, fruit and yogurt.

5. Eat 3 meals and 3 shakes a day. The 3 shakes can be low carb protein shakes. This maintains a steady flow of nutrients for fat loss and muscle growth.

6. Men burn more calories at rest than women, so they have to work less.

7. Eat no carbohydrates and fruits after 5pm. Your body burns carbohydrates and sugars in the morning and stores them as bodyfat at night. Eat protein, fats, and vegetables after 5pm.

Women

1. Figure out your basal metabolic rate (BMR) and make sure it matches your caloric intake. If you are eating you close to your caloric intake and feel full, do not add extra calories. For faster fat loss stay 200-300 calories below your BMR.

2. Drink 8-12 glasses of water a day.

3. Eat or have a snack every 2.5-3 hours. This maintains homeostasis in your body.

4. Snacks can by nuts, chia seeds, protein shakes, protein bars, cheese, beef jerky, fruit and yogurt.

5. Eat 3 meals and 2-3 shakes a day. The 2-3 shakes can be low carb protein shakes. This maintains a steady flow of nutrients for fat loss and muscle growth.

6. Women burn less calories at rest then men. This means they have to work harder to burn fat. So they must do longer cardio sessions if their goal is fat loss.

7. Eat no carbohydrates and fruits after 5pm. Your body burns carbohydrates and sugars in the morning and stores them as bodyfat at night. Eat protein, fats, and vegetables after 5pm.

If your goal is to gain muscle and size, then follow these guidelines.

MEN

1. Figure out your BMR(basal metabolic rate). Match your caloric intake with your BMR. Add extra 800-900 calories per day.

- total caloric intake for the week 800x 7 = 5600 extra calories

2. Drink 8-12 glasses of water a day.

3. Eat or have a snack every 2.5-3 hours. This maintains homeostasis in your body.

4. Snacks can by nuts, chia seeds, protein shakes, protein bars, cheese, beef jerky, fruit and yogurt.

5. Eat 3 meals and 3 shakes a day. The 3 shakes can be weight gainer shakes. This maintains a steady flow of nutrients for and muscle growth and size.

6. Eat calorie dense foods that will feed your muscles for growth. An example of a calorie dense meal would be meat lasagne with a salad. This type of meal is great for weight gain and gaining muscle.

WOMEN

1. Figure out your BMR(basal metabolic rate). Match your caloric intake with your BMR. Add extra 400-500 calories per day.

- total caloric intake for the week 500 x 7 = 3500 extra calories

2. Drink 8-12 glasses of water a day.

3. Eat or have a snack every 3 hours. This maintains homeostasis in your body.

4. Snacks can by nuts, chia seeds, protein shakes, protein bars, cheese, beef jerky, fruit and yogurt.

5. Eat 3 meals and 2 shakes a day. The 2 shakes can be weight gainer shakes. This maintains a steady flow of nutrients for fat loss and muscle growth.

6. Eat calorie dense foods that will feed your muscles for growth. An example of a calorie dense meal would be meat lasagne with a salad. This type of meal is great for weight gain and gaining muscle.

DUMBBELL EXERCISE DESCRIPTIONS

Here are thirty-four exercise descriptions to help you execute proper form. I have included pictures for each exercise. Proper form is the number one priority here. Once you have mastered the form, you can increase the weights.

BACK EXERCISES

1. One Arm Rows

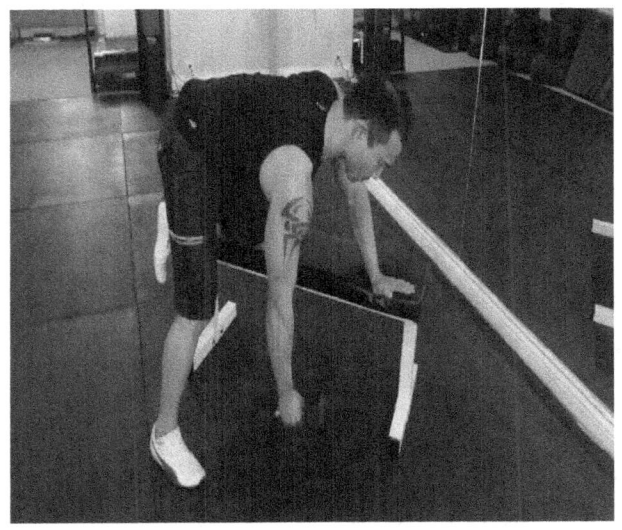 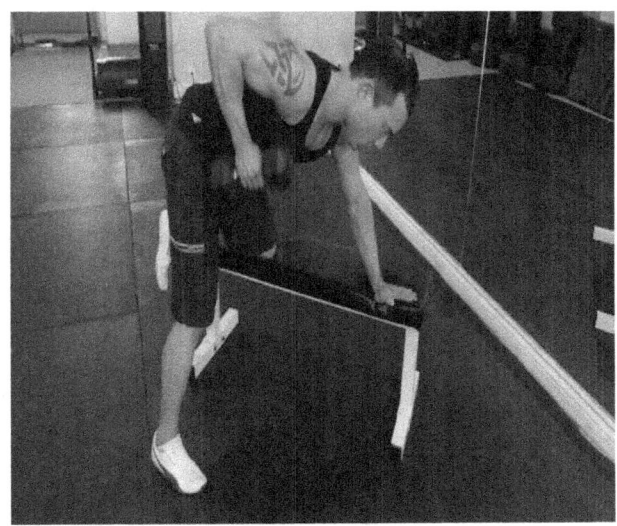

Muscles worked - upper back

Instructions: With right knee and hand on bench with your face looking down. Your back should be straight throughout the movement. Lift the dumbbell to chest/stomach level and lower the weight. Repeat for the other side.

2. Deadlifts

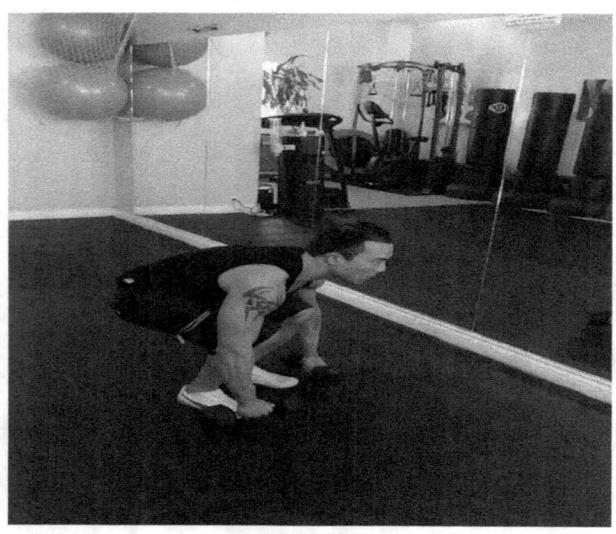 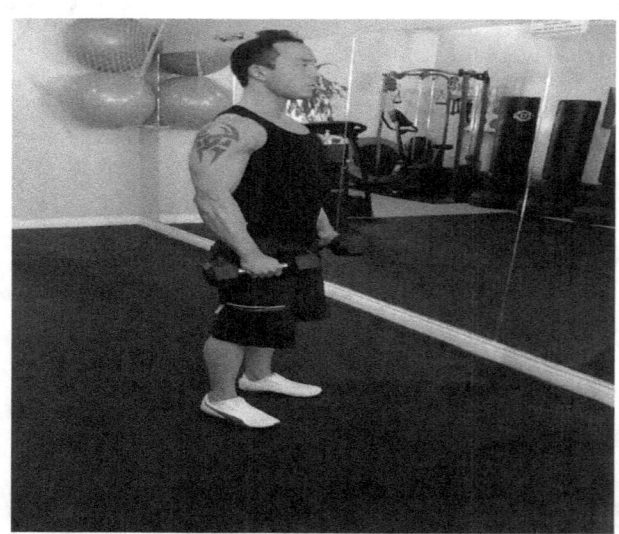

Muscles worked - low/upper back

Instructions: Standing tall with feet shoulder width apart and slightly bent. Lower the dumbbells until they reach the ground if possible. Always keeping your back straight drive with your heels and stand upright. If you can't touch the ground go to your shins.

3. Push-Up To Rows

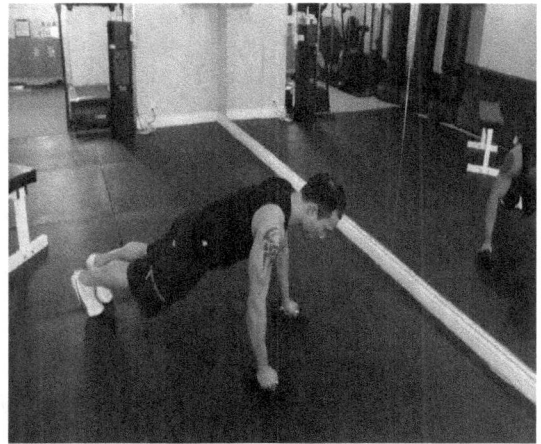 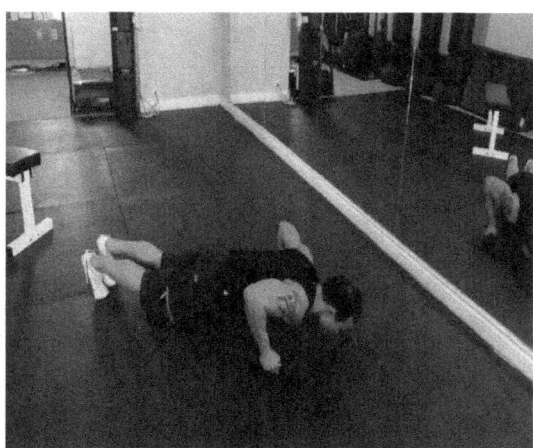

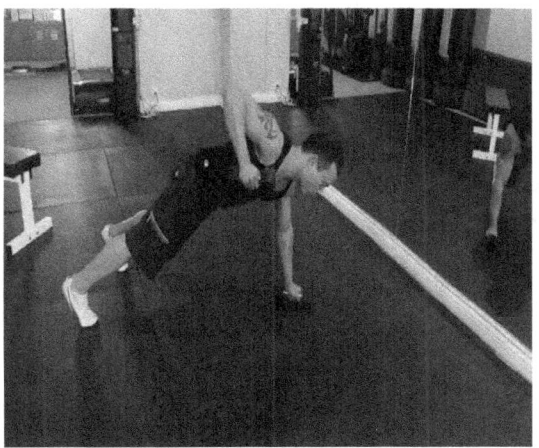 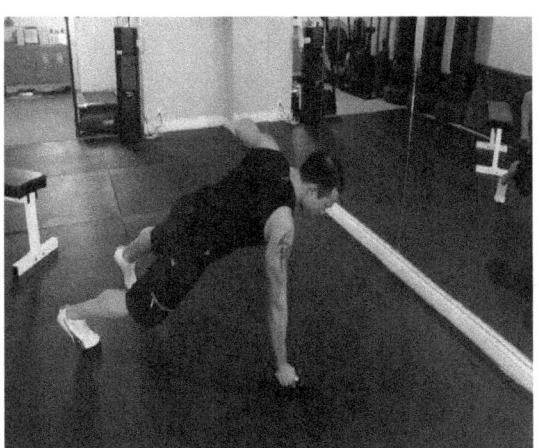

Muscles worked - chest/back/core

Instructions: This is an advanced movement and not for beginners. In a push-up position with 2 dumbbells underneath you palms facing each other. Feet should be shoulder width apart and in a plank position. Do a push up then lift one dumbbell up to your chest and return it to the ground. Stay in a plank position and repeat for the other side.

4. Bent Over Rows

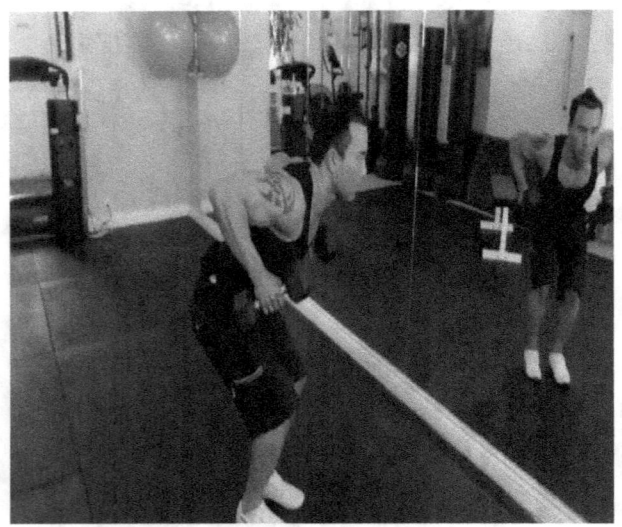 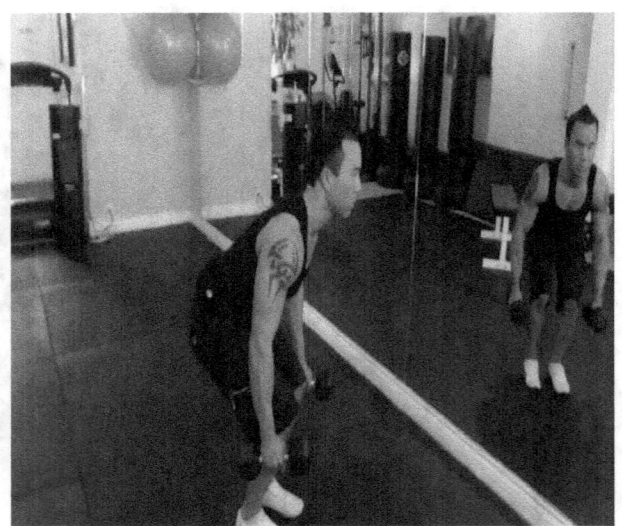

Muscles worked - upper back
Instructions: Bent over on angle with dumbbells in hand with back straight. Lift dumbbells up to your chest and squeeze your shoulder blades together for maximum contraction. Return to starting position and repeat.

CHEST

5. Flat Bench Press

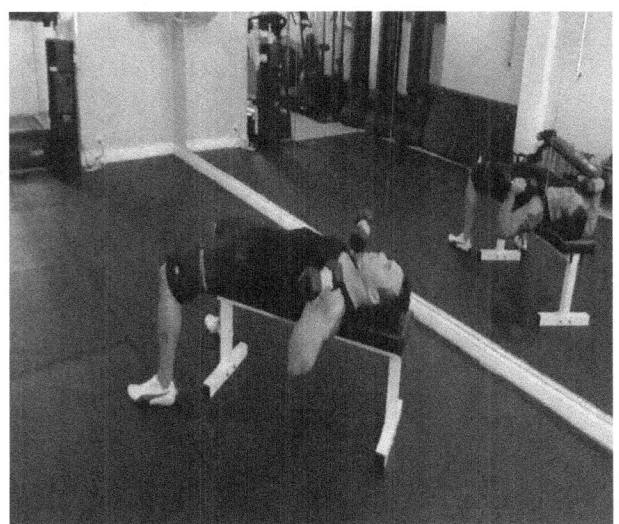 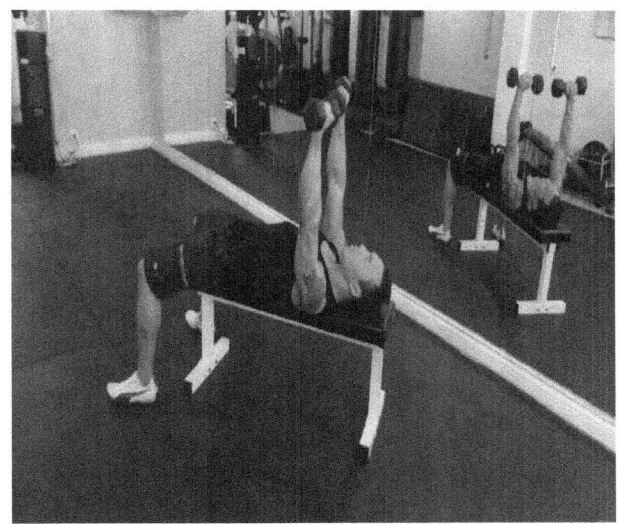

Muscles worked - middle chest

Instructions: Lie on the bench with feet flat on the ground. If your a female you can put your feet on the bench to protect your arch. Starting point should be at chest level with elbows out by side. Lift dumbbells into the air but do not lock out your elbows and return to starting position.

6. Incline Bench Press

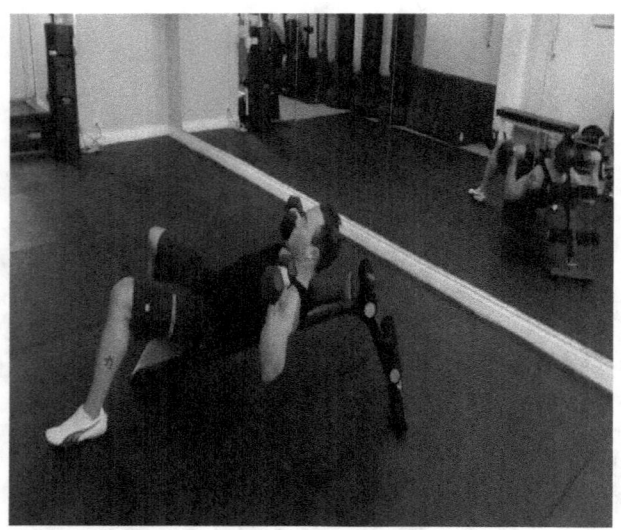 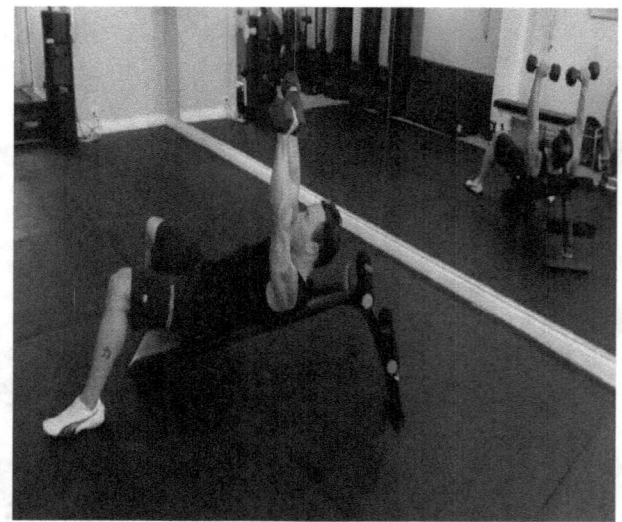

Muscles worked - upper chest
Instructions: Lie on a bench with an incline upwards. With both feet planted on the ground lift both dumbbells into the air but do not lock out your elbows. Return to starting position and repeat.

7. Decline Bench Press

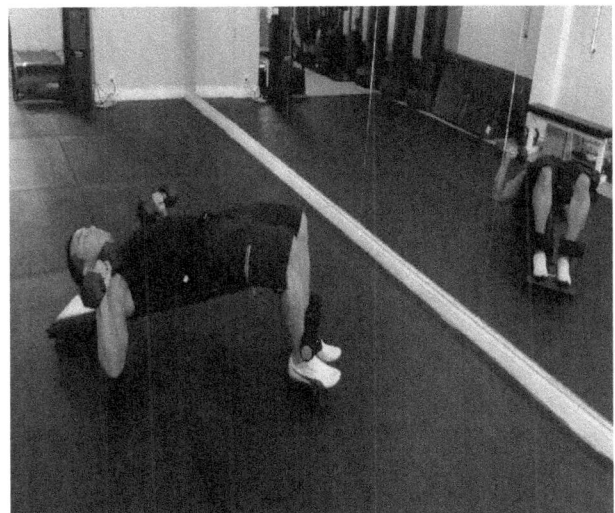 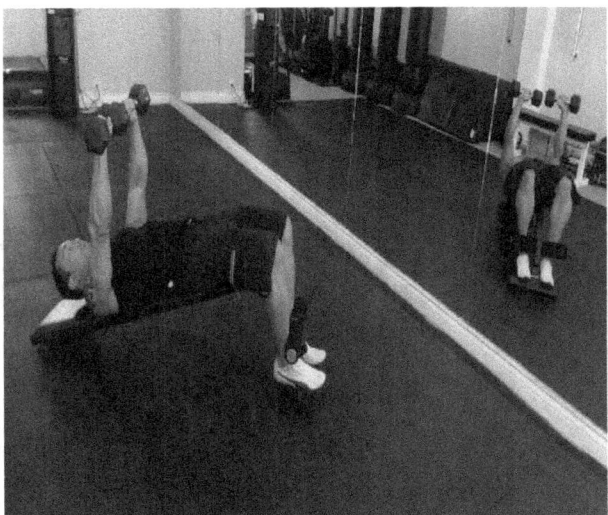

Muscles worked - middle and lower chest
Instructions: Lie on a bench on a decline downwards. Your legs can be on the bench or feet locked under the pads. Lift dumbbells upwards without locking out elbows and return to starting position.

8. Incline Fly

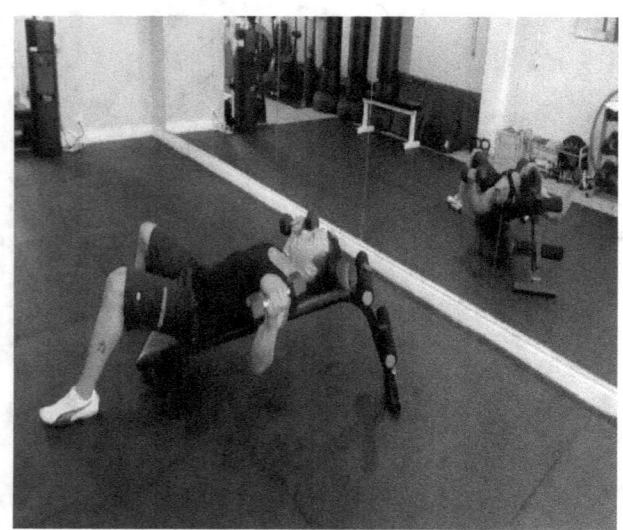 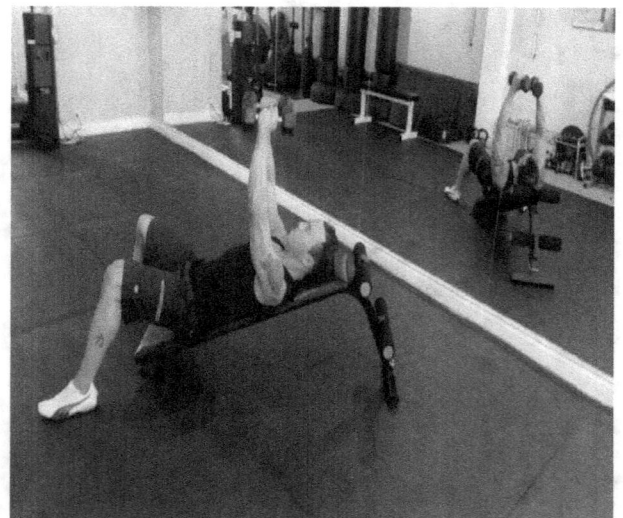

Muscles worked - upper and outer chest
Instructions: Lie on a bench with an upward incline. Dumbbells should be over you head with elbows bent. Lower dumbbells in a controlled manner and return to starting position.

9. Flat Fly

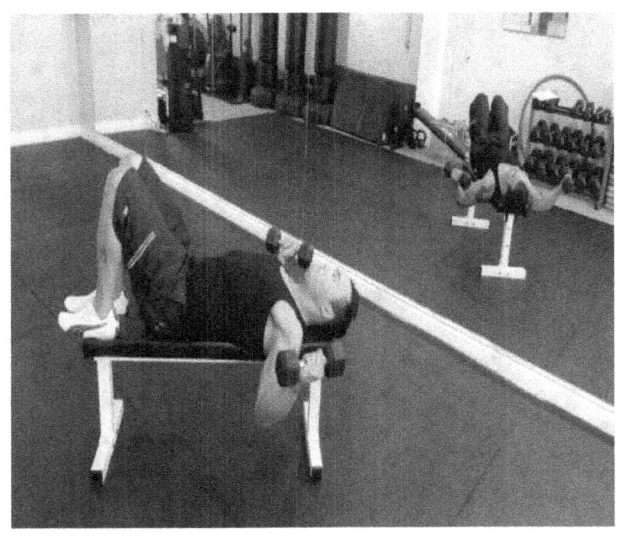 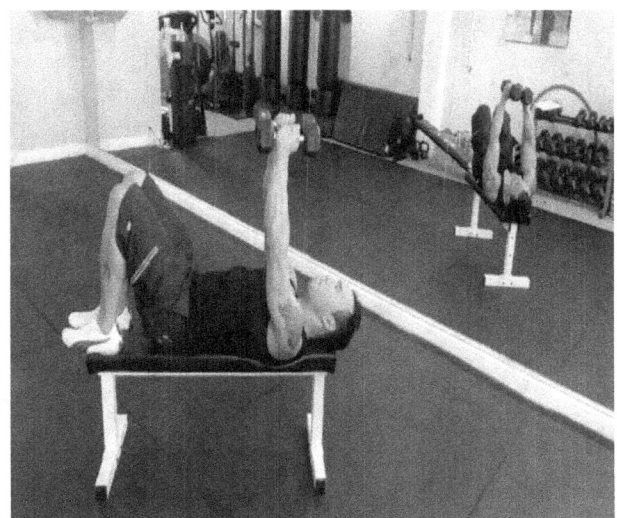

Muscles worked - middle and outer chest
Instructions: Lie on a bench with both feet flat. Dumbbells should be over your chest with elbows bent. Lower the dumbbells slowly and return to starting position.

10. Decline Fly

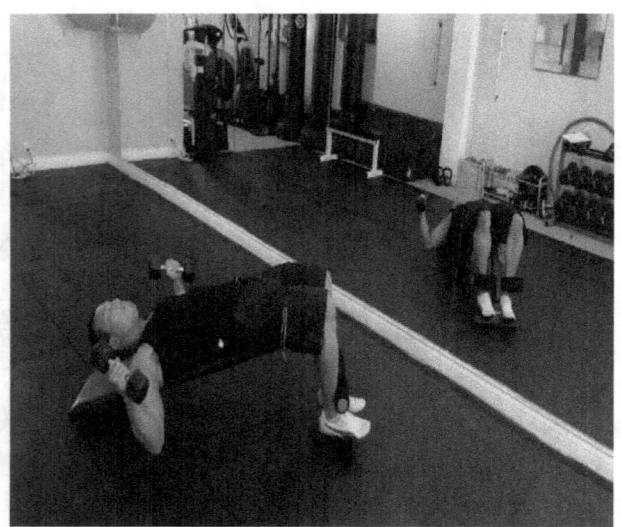 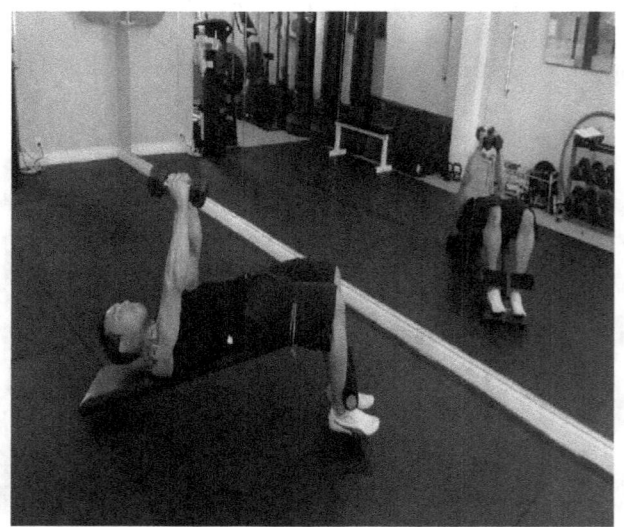

Muscles worked - lower and outer chest
Instructions: Lie on a bench with a downward decline. Dumbbells should be above you with elbows bent slightly. Lower in a controlled manner and return to starting position.

11. Dumbbell Pullovers

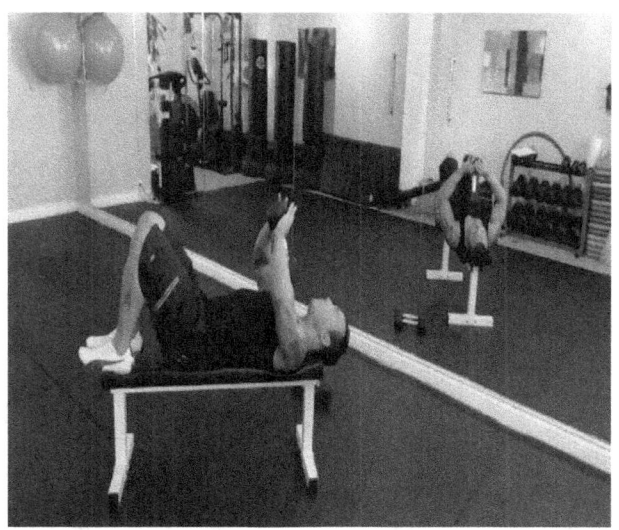 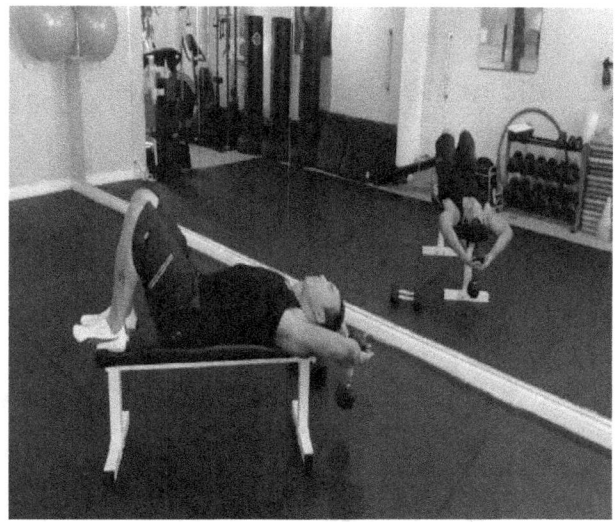

Muscles worked - outer chest/back

Instructions: Lie on your back with feet flat on the ground or bench. Holding the top of the dumbbell over your head with arms bent slightly. Lower the dumbbell until your get a really good stretch in your chest/lats and then return to starting position.

QUADRICEPS

12. Holding Dumbbell Squats

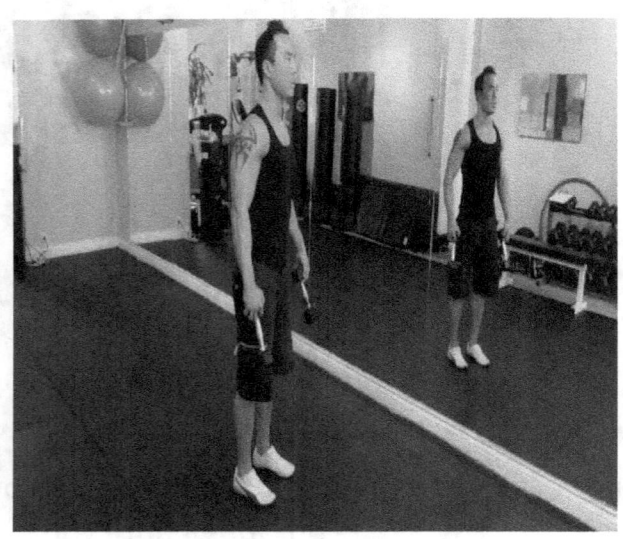 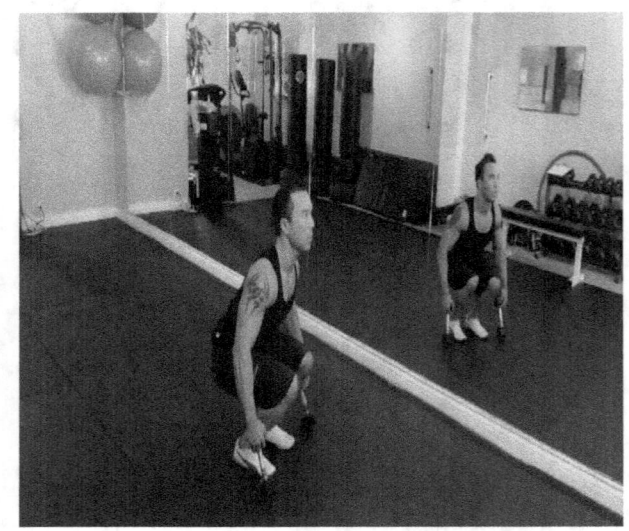

Muscles worked - quadriceps
Instructions: Keeping feet shoulder width apart with dumbbells at side. Lower the dumbbells until they touch the floor or go as low as you can. Keep your core tight throughout the movement and return to staring position.

13. Front Squats

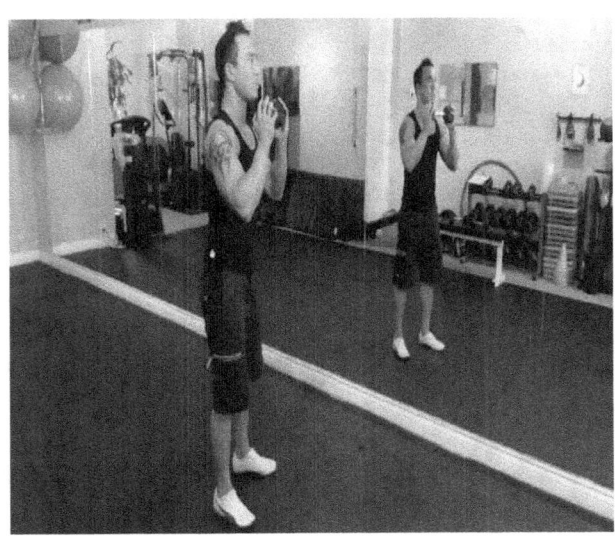 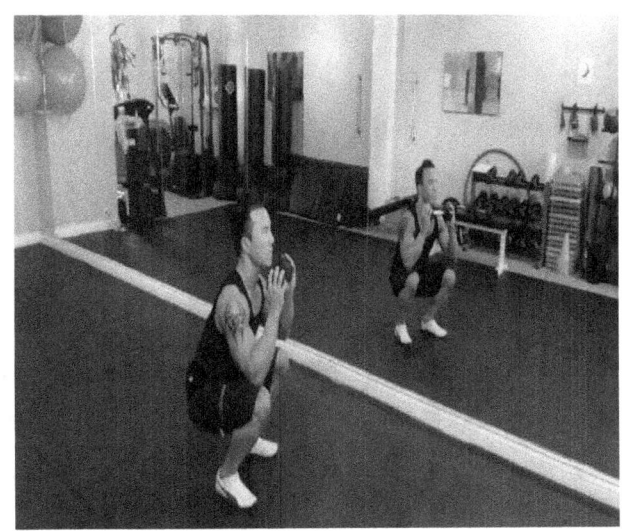

Muscles worked - quadriceps

Instructions: Keeping feet shoulder width apart holding dumbbell in front of face. Squat and go as low as you can without breaking proper form. Do half squats first to build up your hip flexors then graduate to full squats.

14. Plie Squats

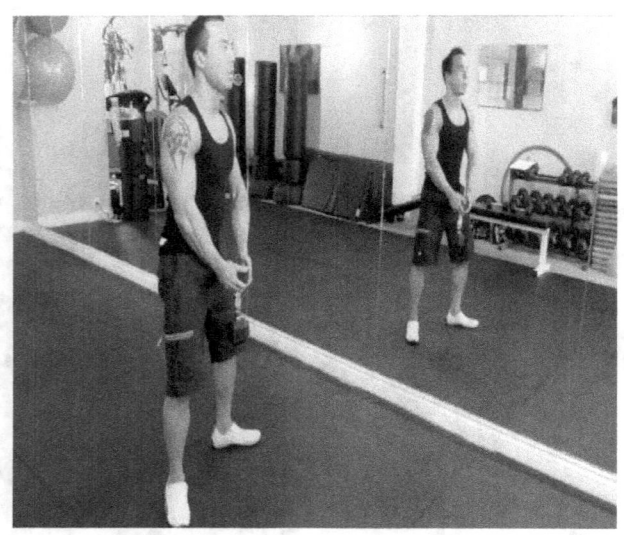 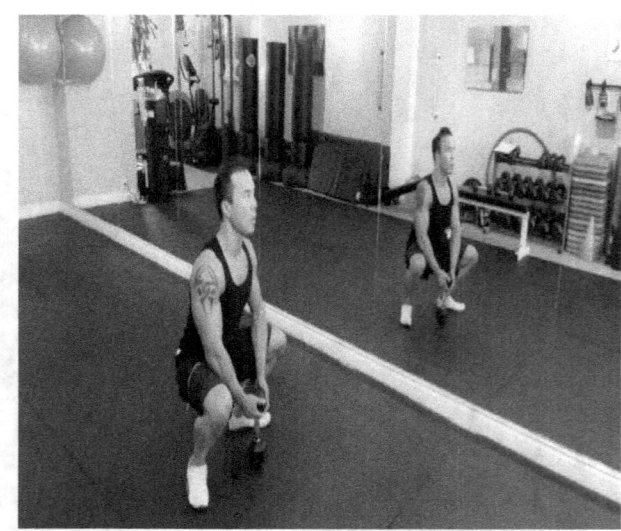

Muscles worked - inner quadriceps

Instructions: Start by standing feet shoulder width apart but feet turned outwards like in a plie stance. Do a squat and go as low as you can without bending forward or breaking form. Return to starting position and repeat.

15. V-up Leg Extensions

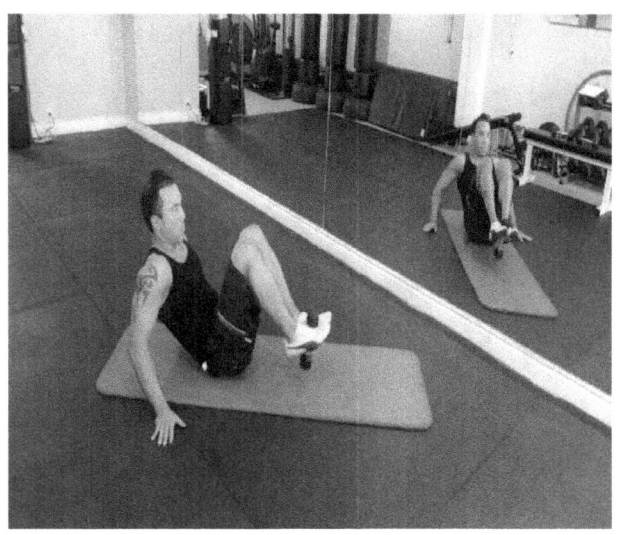 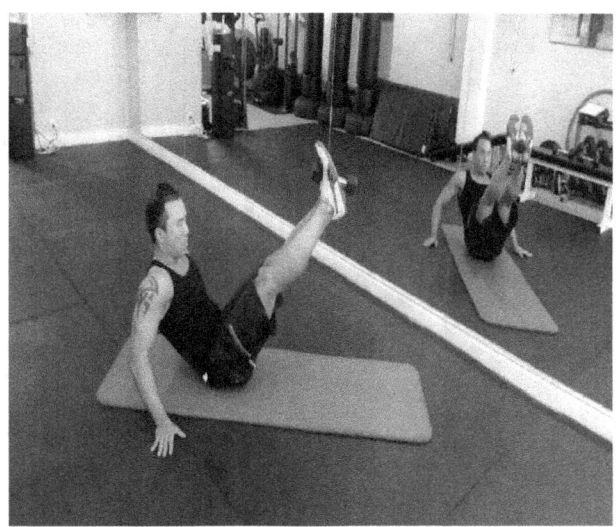

Muscles worked – quadriceps/core

Instructions: This is more an advanced exercise. Start by putting a dumbbell between your feet and in a v-up position. Extend your legs until your quads contract then return to starting position and repeat. Best to use a light weight to start.

16. Split Squats

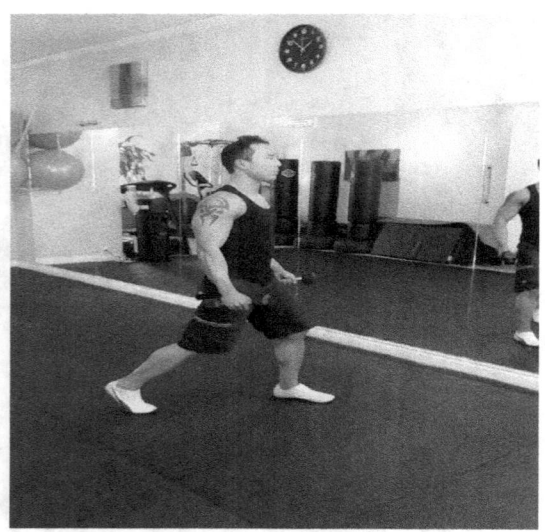 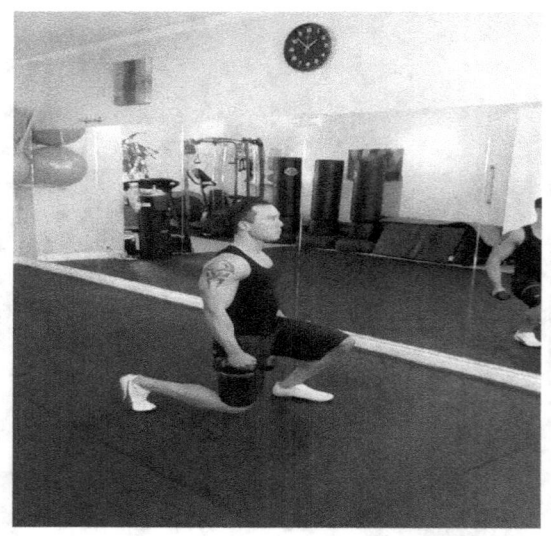

Muscles worked – quadriceps/glutes

Instructions: Starting with feet shoulder width apart and holding dumbbells at side. Bring your right foot back 3 steps back. Standing on your right upper foot and and left foot flat, bring your right knee towards the ground but do not hit your knee on the ground. Return to starting position and repeat for the other leg. Keep your body upright throughout the movement.

HAMSTRINGS

17. One Legged Deadlifts

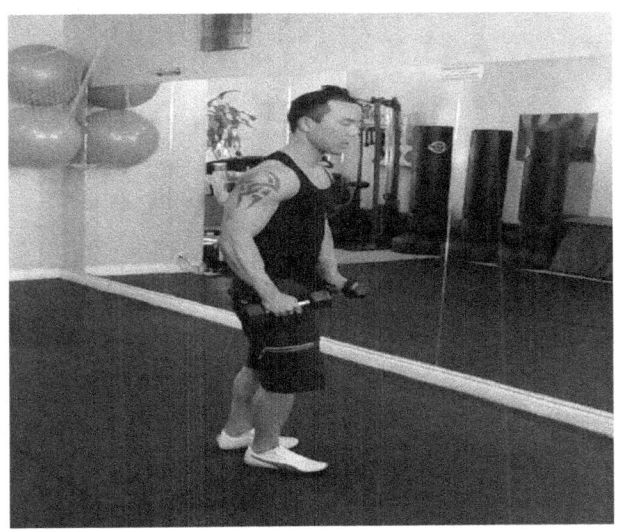 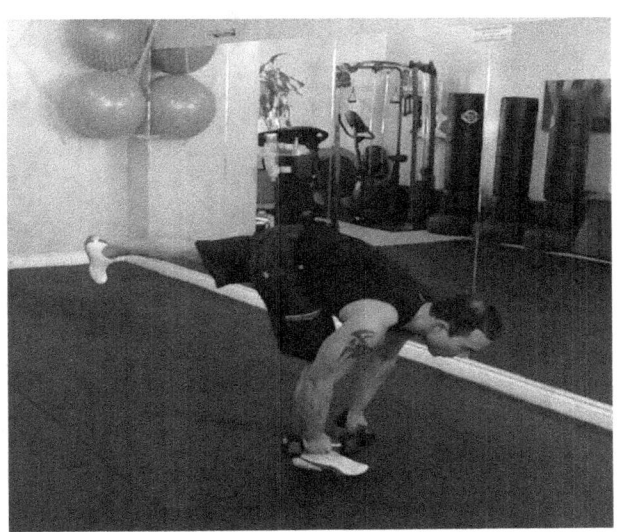

Muscles worked - hamstrings/low back
Instructions: Standing with feet shoulder width apart and 2 dumbbells close to your left leg. Slowly let the descend towards the your shin. At the same time your right leg should come in the air until it is parallel to the floor. Repeat for the other side.

18. Stiff Legged Deadlifts

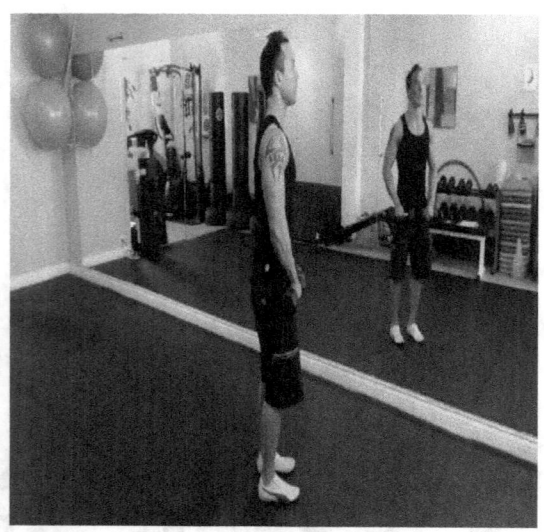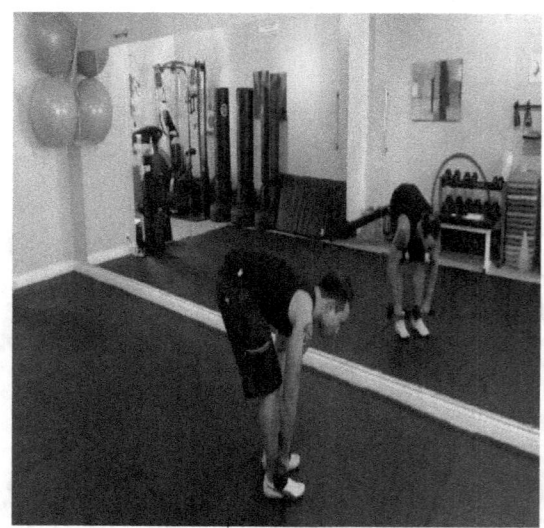

Muscles worked - hamstrings/low back
Instructions: Standing with feet shoulder width apart and knees slightly bent. Slowly let the dumbbells descend and keep them close to your legs and shin. Keep back straight at all times.

19. Lying Leg Curls

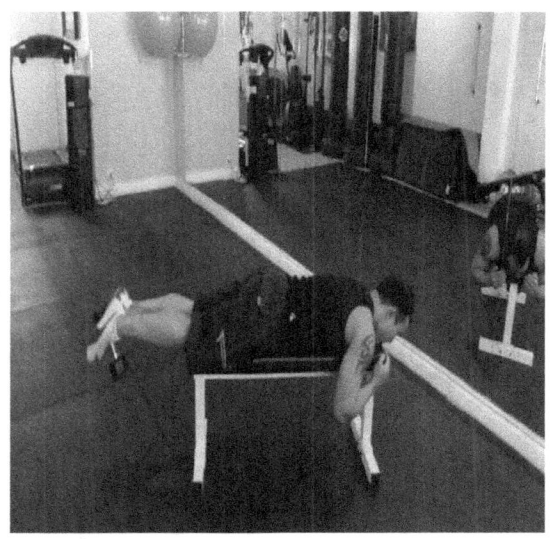 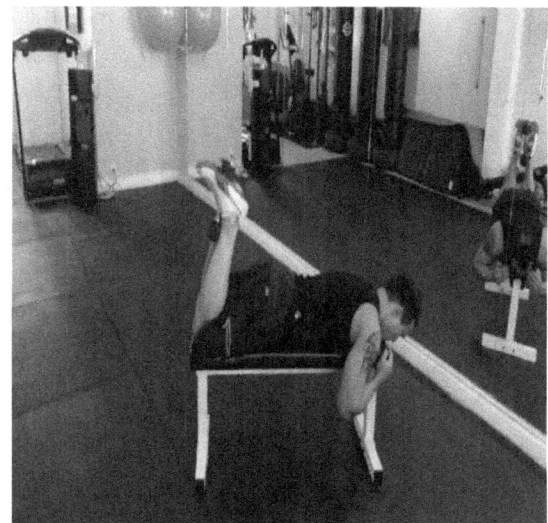

Muscles worked – hamstrings/calves

Instructions: Lying supine position on a bench have a person put a dumbbell between your feet. Your knees should be on the bench for support. Hold the dumbbell and curl it towards your glutes and return to starting position.

HIPS(Abductors/Adductors)

20. Side To Side Lunge - Muscles worked - hips/inner thighs

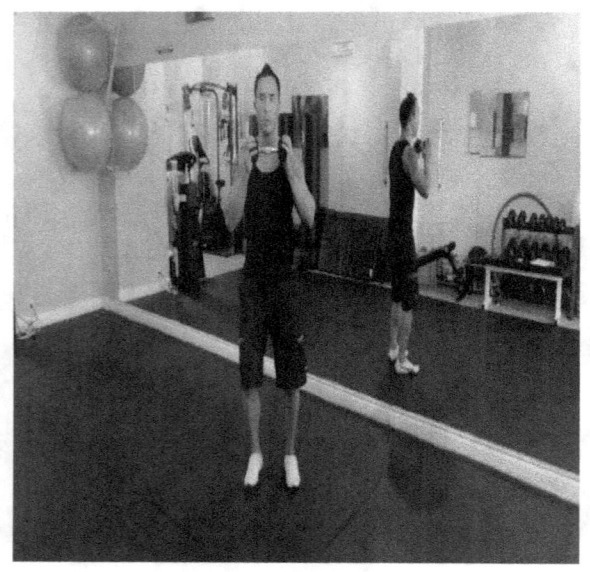
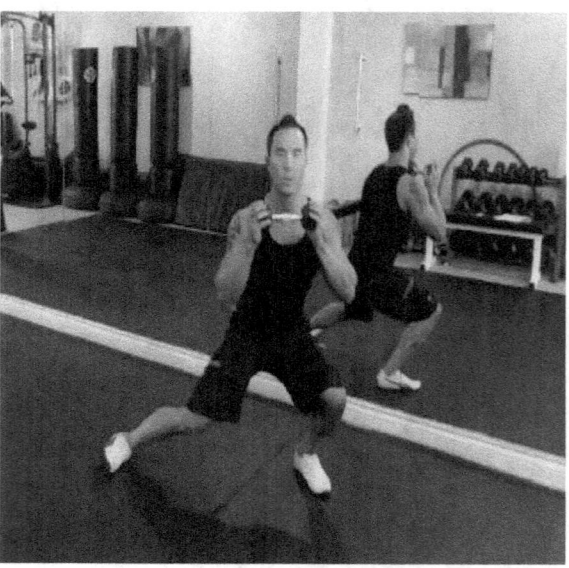
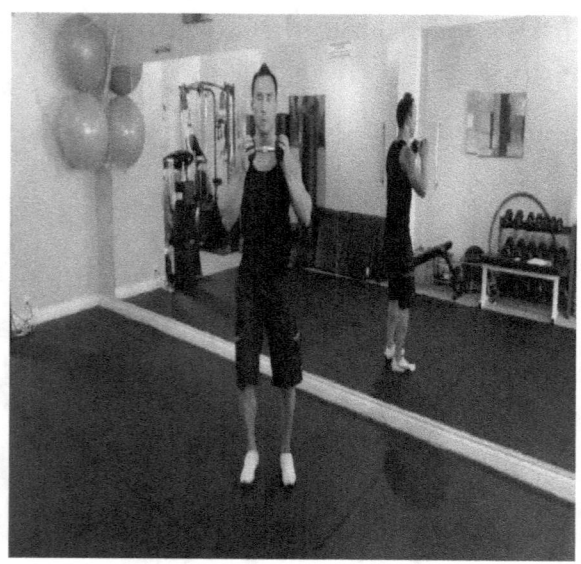
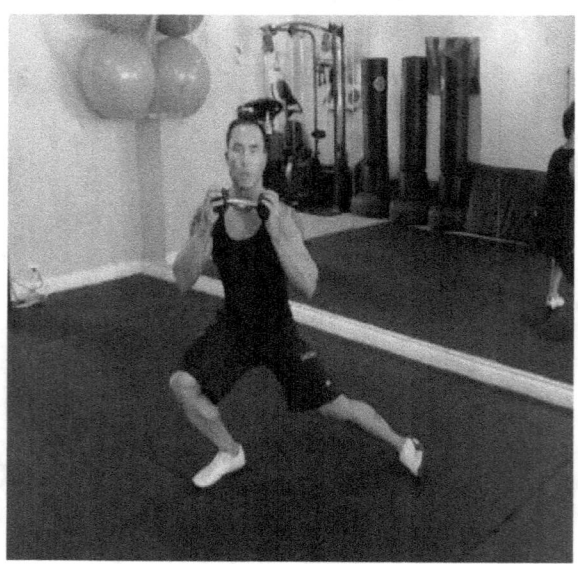

Instructions: Holding a dumbbell in front of your face with feet shoulder width apart. Step sideways with your right leg and keep your left leg straight. Go down as far as you can and repeat for the other side.

SHOULDERS

21. Shoulder Press

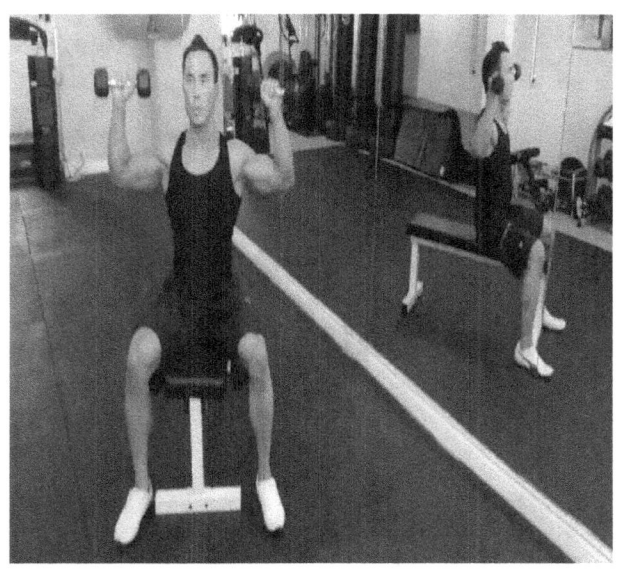 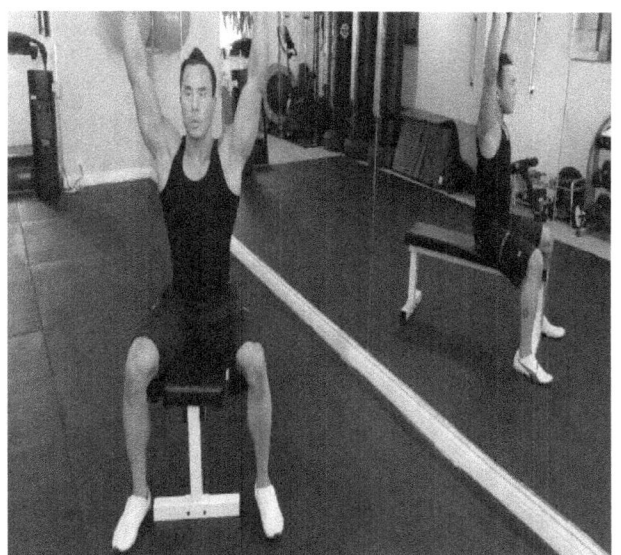

Muscles worked - front/side shoulders
Instructions: Seated on bench with feet flat and back straight. Lift dumbbells upward and do not lock out your elbows. Keep the movement fluid as you press upwards and come downwards.

22. Side Laterals

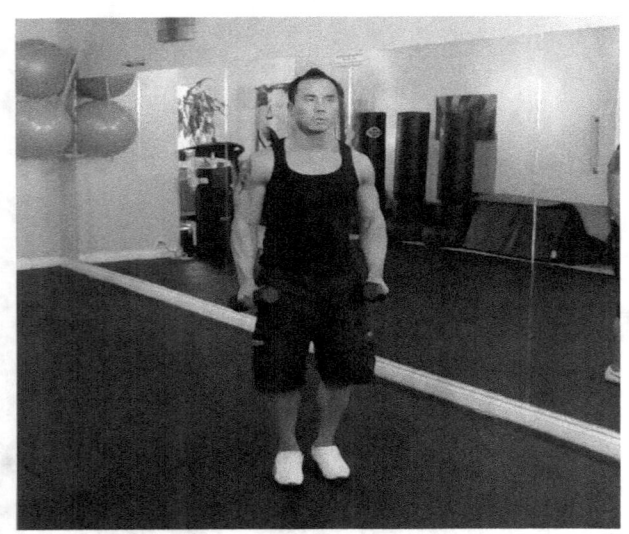 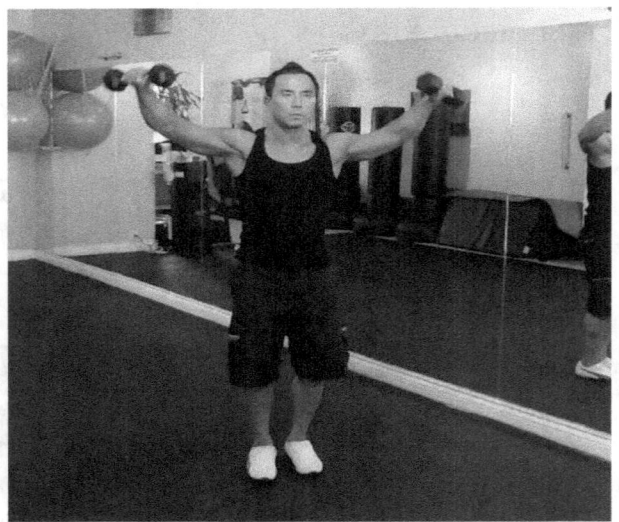

Muscles worked - side shoulders

Instructions: Start by having dumbbells by your side and legs slightly bent. Elbows should be bent slightly throughout the movement. Lift dumbbells upward until they reach shoulder level and return to starting position.

23. Rotation Presses

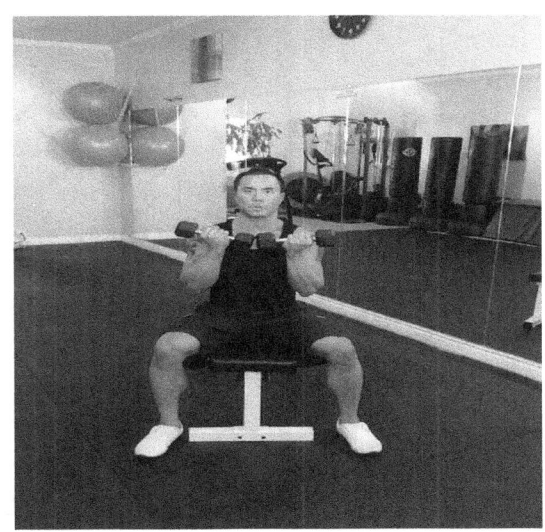 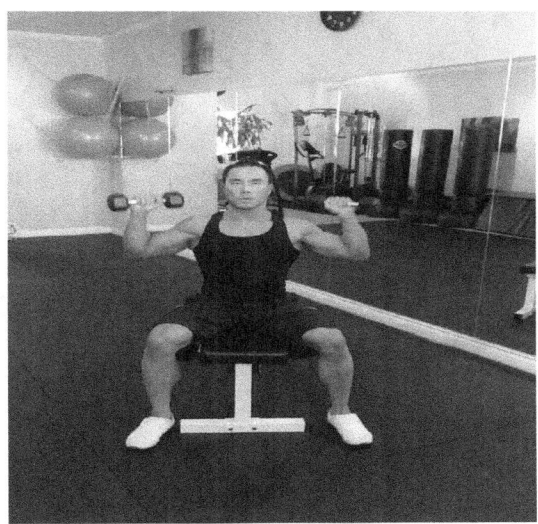

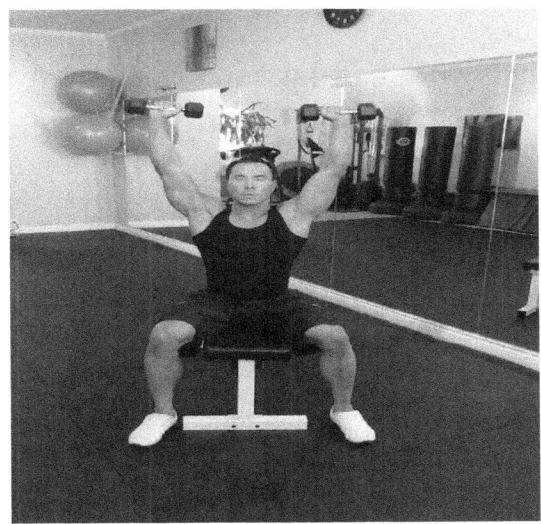

Muscles worked - front/side/rear shoulders
Instructions: Seated on a bench with feet flat and back straight. Hold the 2 dumbbells with palms facing your face rotate the dumbbells outwards and then do a shoulder press. Bring them down and rotate them inwards to starting position.

24. Bent Over Laterals

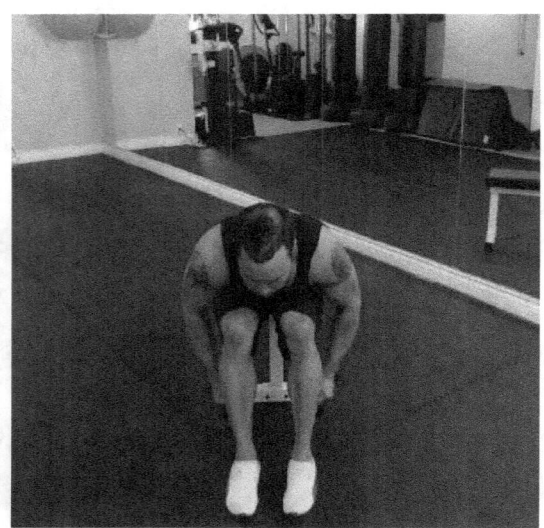 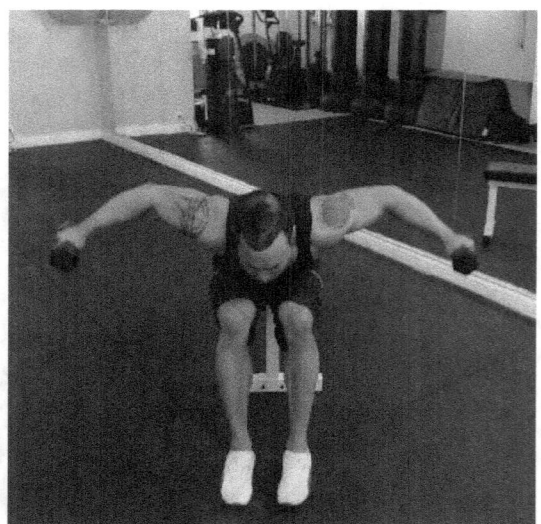

Muscles worked - rear shoulders
Instructions: Seated on a bench with feet flat and back bent over on an angle. Lift dumbbells until the are parallel to the floor. Return to starting position and repeat.

25. Upright Rows

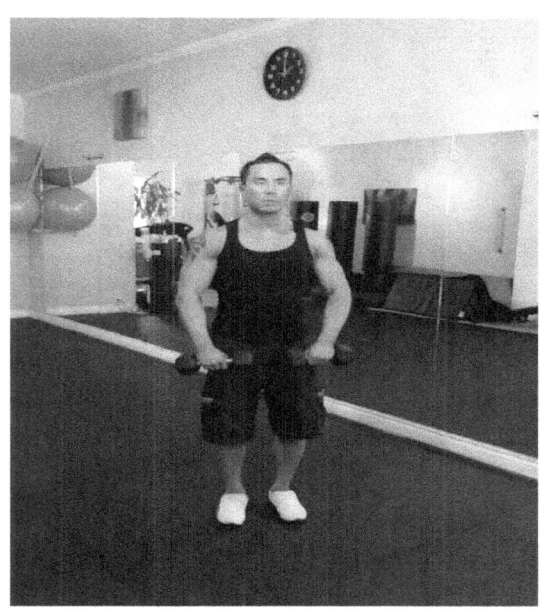 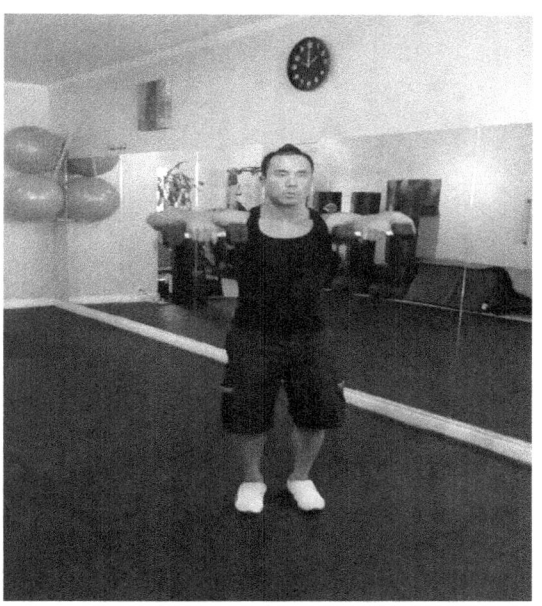

Muscles worked - side delts/traps

Instructions: Standing with feet shoulder width apart and knees slightly bent. Lift both dumbbells upwards until they are at chest level. Your elbows should be flared out at end position.

CALVES

26. Calf Rocks

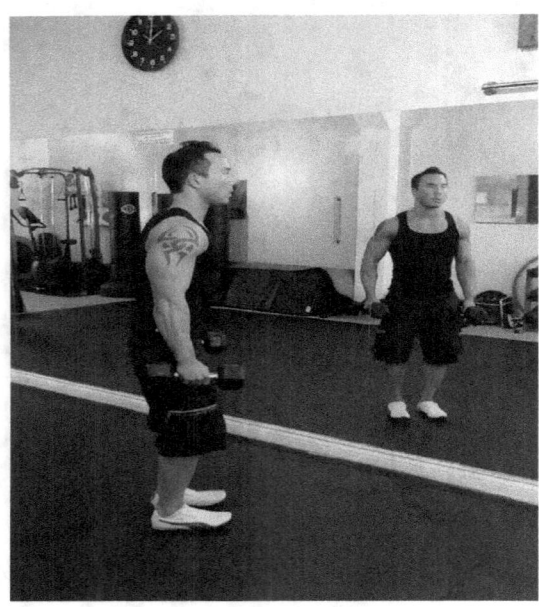 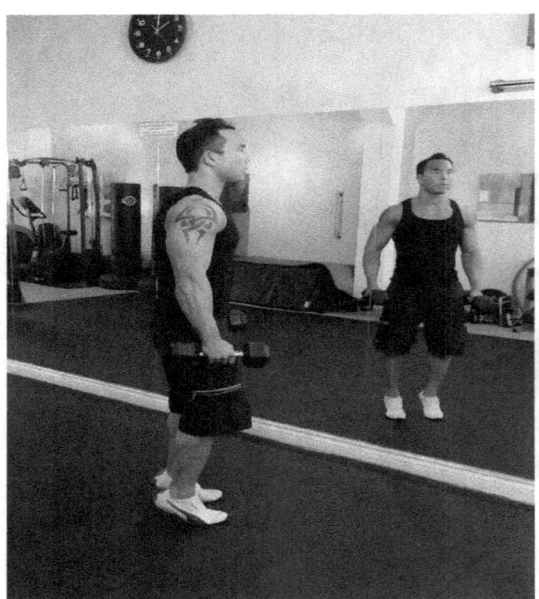

Muscles worked - front/rear calves
Instructions: Standing with feet shoulder width apart and keeping eyes forward. Knees slightly bent rock forward onto your toes and rock backwards onto your heels. Keep the motion fluid.

27. One Legged Calf Raises

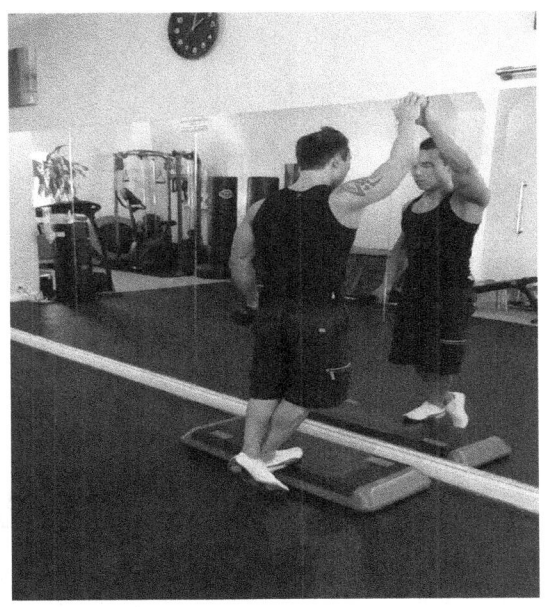 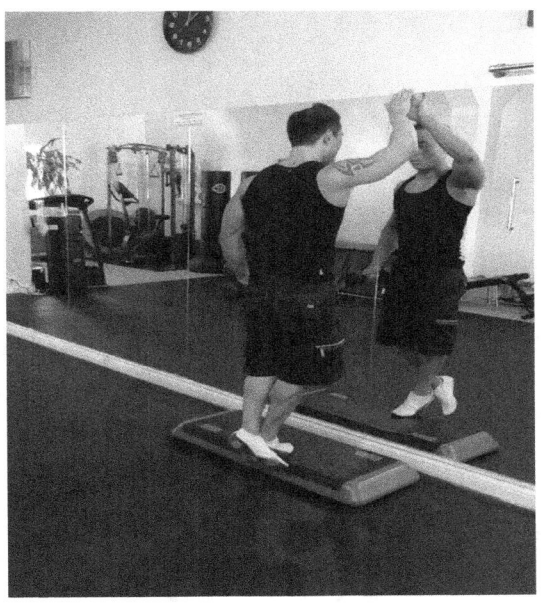

Muscles worked - rear calves

Instructions: Using stairs or a platform hold one dumbbell in one hand and use the other one for balance. Push off with your toes and then return to starting position. Repeat for other side.

TRICEPS

28. Overhead Extension

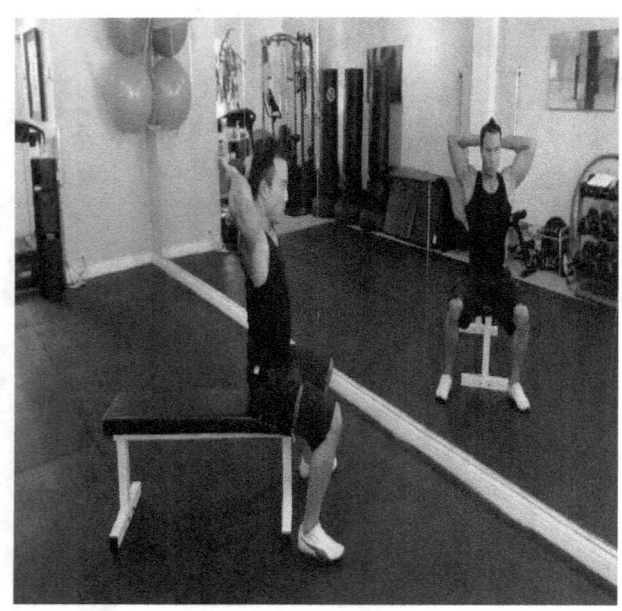 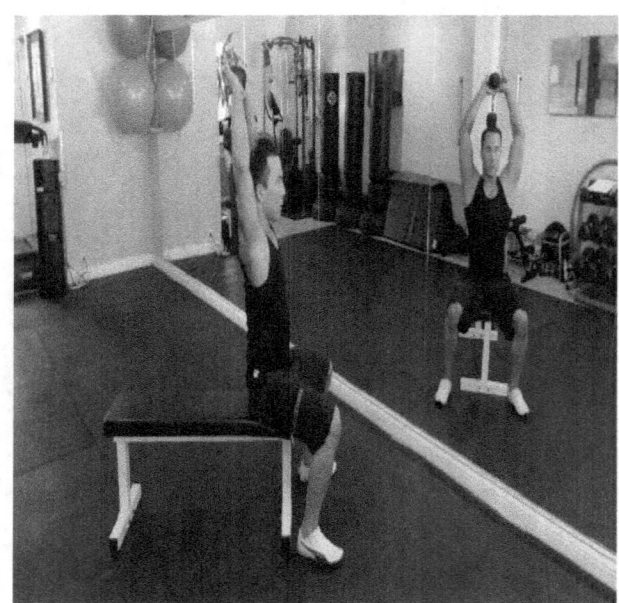

Muscles worked - triceps

Instructions: Seated on a bench with feet flat. Holding one dumbbell with both hands in the air above your head. Lower the dumbbell behind your head and return to starting position but do not lock out your elbows. Keep back straight throughout the movement.

29. One Arm Kickbacks

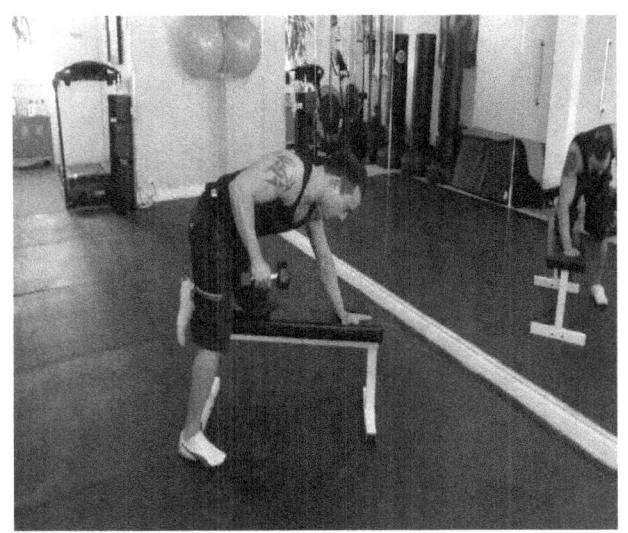 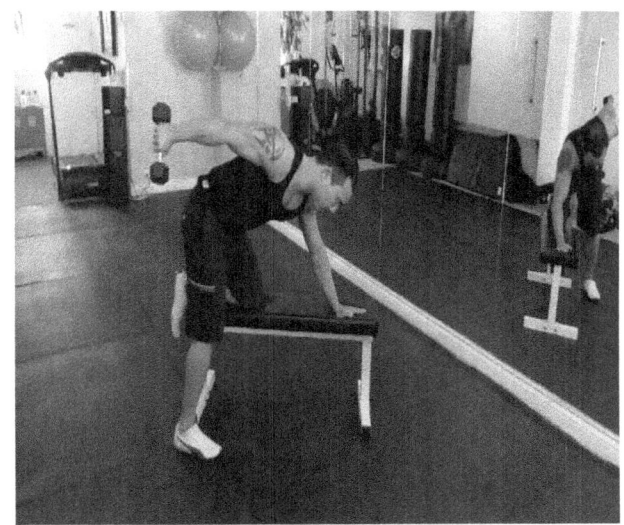

Muscles worked - triceps

Instructions: With right knee and hand on the bench and keeping neck straight. Lift dumbbell upwards and return to starting position. Repeat for the other side.

30. Lying Extensions

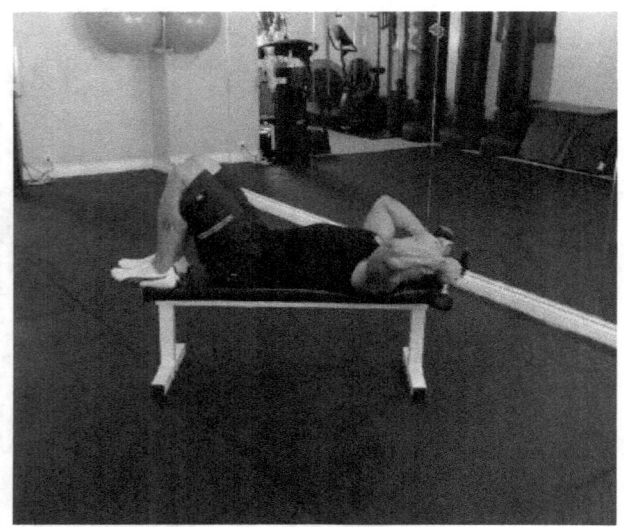 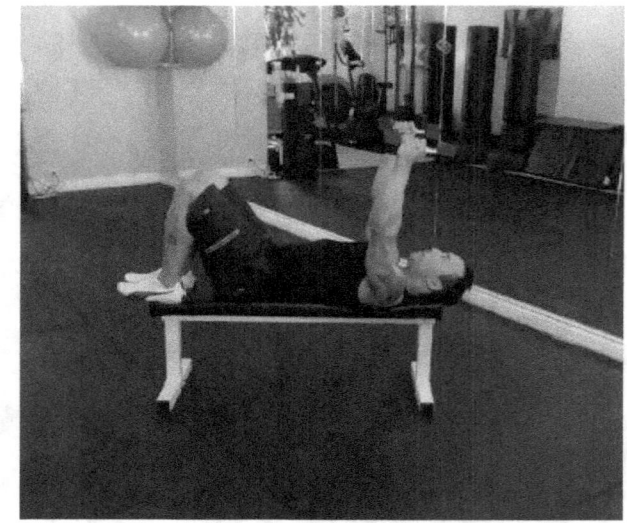

Muscles worked - triceps
Instructions: Lying on the bench with feet on the bench or on the floor. With 2 dumbbells above your head palms facing each other. Let dumbbells slowly descend then return to starting position.

31. Bench Dips

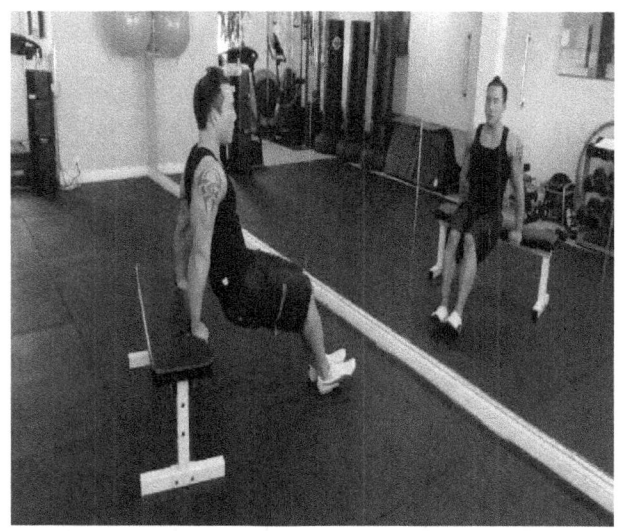 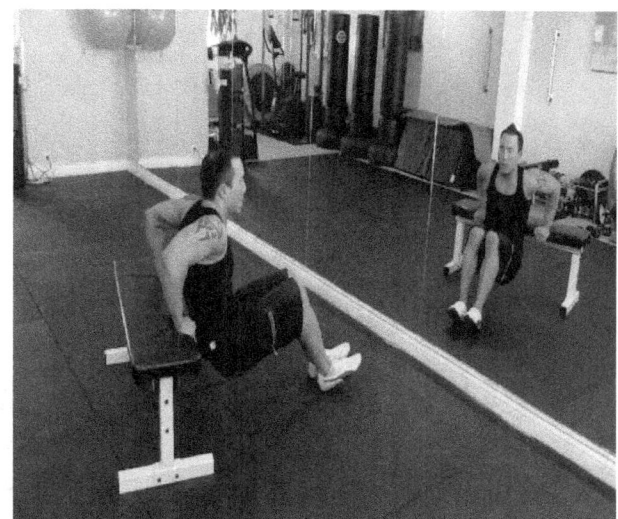

Muscles worked – triceps/shoulders
Instructions: Both hands on bench with knees bent with feet flat. Legs can be straight or further for more resistance. Descend slowly until arms are bent and then return to starting position.

BICEPS

32. Alternate Curls

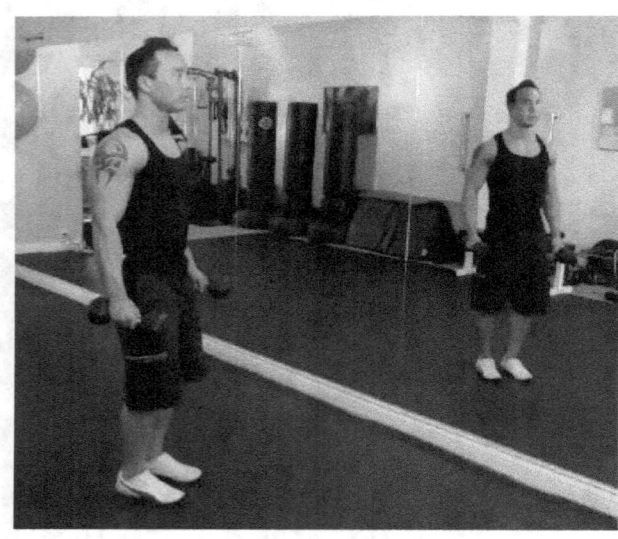 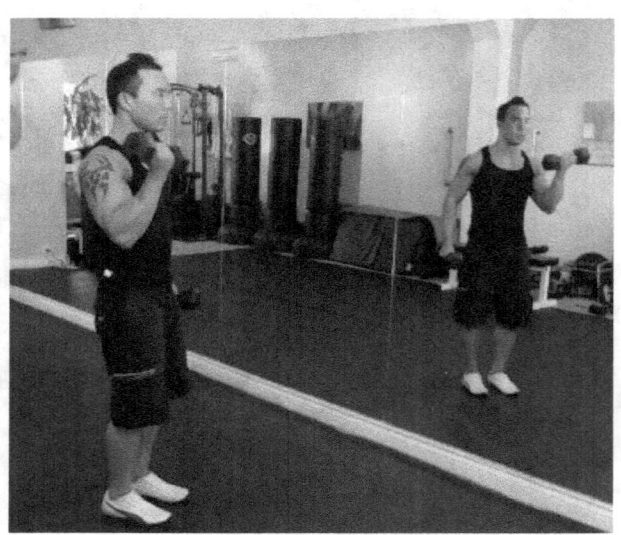

Muscles worked - biceps
Instructions: Standing tall but knees slightly bent. Simply supinate one dumbbell upwards but stop before your shoulder. Return to starting position and repeat for the other side.

33. Hammer Curls

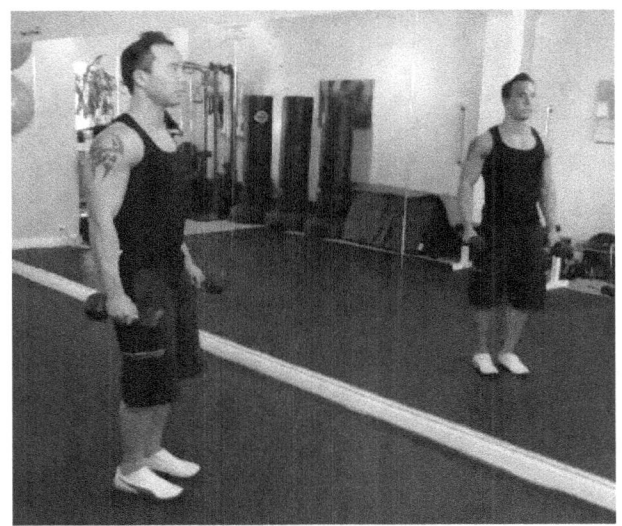 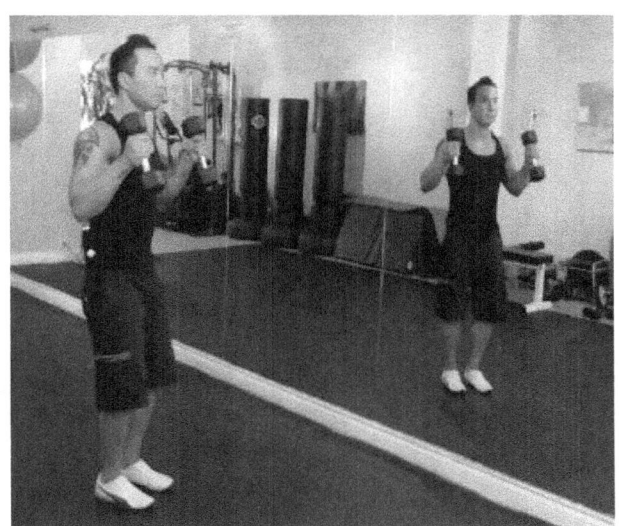

Muscles worked - biceps/forearms
Instructions: Standing with knees slightly bent and palms facing inward. Lift both dumbbells upwards but stop before you reach the shoulders and return to starting position.

34. Once Arm Concentration Curls

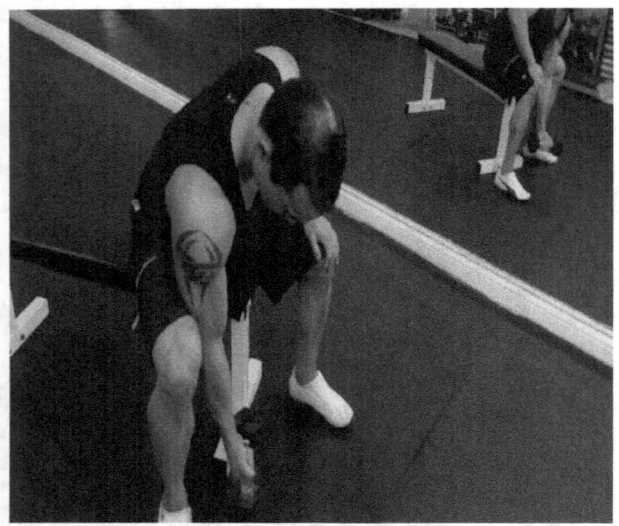 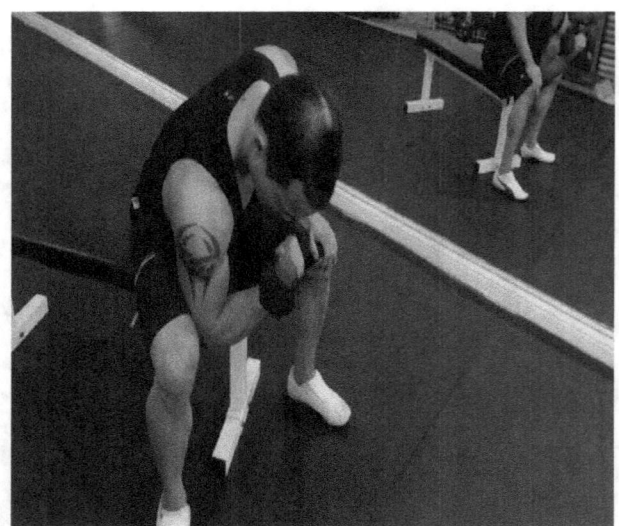

Muscles worked - biceps

Instructions: Seated on the end of a bench bent over with one dumbbell in hand. Elbow is against your inner thigh for support. Lift dumbbell upwards and squeeze the biceps and return to starting position. Repeat for other side.

DUMBBELL WORKOUTS FOR MEN

Some guys like to grunt while they train. I never understood why they like to do this. I prefer to reserve my energy for the next set. If you have to grunt or yell, do it in your basement, not at the gym. The girls are not impressed. Here are eight dumbbell workouts for men. Bring on the sweat!

Two Beginner Workouts

Workout 1 – Level 1

1. Warm up for 5-6 minutes

2. Exercise 1 - one arm dumbbell rows – 1x12, 1x10, 1x8 reps

3. Exercise 14 - plie squats – 1x12, 1x10, 1x8 reps

4. Exercise 5 - bench press flat – 1x12, 1x10, 1x8 reps

5. Running on spot for 1 minute

6. Exercise 18 - stiff legged dead lifts – 1x12, 1x10, 1x8 reps

7. Exercise 26 - calf rocks – 1x20, 1x20, 1x20 reps

8. Exercise 21 - shoulder press – 1x12, 1x10, 1x8 reps

9. Exercise 31 - bench dips – 1x14, 1x10, 1x8 reps

10. Exercise 34 - one arm concentration curls – 1x12, 1x10, 1x8 reps

11. Cool down for 5-6 minutes

12. Static stretching

Workout 2 – Level 1

1. Warm up for 5-6 minutes

2. Exercise 2 - dead lifts – 1x10, 1x8, 1x6 reps

3. Exercise 13 - front squats – 1x10, 1x8, 1x6 reps

4. Exercise 8 - incline fly – 1x10, 1x8, 1x6 reps

5. Jumping jacks – 1x20, 1x20, 1x20 reps

6. Exercise 19 – lying leg curls - 1x10, 1x8, 1x6 reps

7. Exercise 24 - bent over laterals - 1x10, 1x8, 1x6 reps

8. Exercise 20 - side to side lunge – 1x10, 1x10, 1x10 reps

9. Cool down for 5-6 minutes

10. Static stretching

Two Intermediate Workouts

Workout 1 – Level 2

1. Warm up for 5-6 minutes

2. Exercise 12 - holding dumbbell squats – 1x12, 1x10, 1x8, 1x6 reps

3. Exercise 4 - bent over rows - 1x12, 1x10, 1x8, 1x6 reps for each side

4. Running on spot – 1x30, 1x30, 1x30 seconds

5. Exercise 9 - flat fly - 1x12, 1x10, 1x8, 1x6 reps

6. Exercise 27 - one legged calf raises – 1x20, 1x18, 1x16, 1x14 reps for each side

7. Exercise 25 - upright row - 1x12, 1x10, 1x8, 1x6 reps

8. Exercise 28 - overhead extensions - 1x12, 1x10, 1x8, 1x6 reps

9. Exercise 33 - hammer curls - 1x12, 1x10, 1x8, 1x6 reps

10. Cool down - 5-6 minutes

11. Static stretching

Workout 2 – Level 2

1. Warm up for 5-6 minutes

2. Exercise 11 - pullovers – 1x10, 1x8, 1x6, 1x4 reps

3. Exercise 15 - V-up leg extensions - 1x12, 1x10, 1x8, 1x6 reps

4. Push-ups – 1x15, 1x15, 1x15, 1x15 reps

5. Jumping jacks – 1x25, 1x25, 1x25, 1x25 reps

6. Exercise 17 - one legged dead lifts - 1x10, 1x8, 1x6, 1x4 reps

7. Exercise 23 - rotation presses - 1x10, 1x8, 1x6, 1x4 reps

8. Cool down - 5-6 minutes

9. Static stretching

Four Advanced Workouts

Workout 1- Level 3

1. Warm up for 5-6 minutes

2. Exercise 2 - dead lifts – 1x10, 1x8, 1x6, 1x4, 1x2 reps

3. Exercise 14 - plie squats - 1x12, 1x10, 1x8, 1x6, 1x4 reps

4. Exercise 3 - push up to rows - 1x10, 1x8, 1x6, 1x4 reps for each side

5. Jumping jacks – 1x30, 1x30, 1x30, 1x30 reps

6. Exercise 21 - shoulder press - 1x10, 1x8, 1x6, 1x4, 1x2 reps

7. Exercise 19 - lying leg curls - 1x10, 1x8, 1x6, 1x4, 1x2 reps

8. Exercise 26 - calf rocks - 1x20, 1x18, 1x16, 1x14, 1x12 reps

9. Exercise 31 - bench dips - 1x25, 1x20, 1x15, 1x10, 1x8 reps

10. Exercise 32 - alternate curls - 1x10, 1x8, 1x6, 1x4, 1x2 reps

11. Cool down for 5 - 6 minutes

12. Static stretching

Workout 2- Level 3

1. Warm up for 5-6 minutes

2. Exercise 11 - pullovers – 1x10, 1x8, 1x6, 1x4, 1x2 reps

3. Exercise 1 - one arm rows - 1x10, 1x8, 1x6, 1x4, 1x2 reps

4. Super set exercise 2 and 3 together *

5. Exercise 15 - v-up leg extensions -1x12, 1x10, 1x8, 1x6, 1x4 reps

6. Exercise 16 - split squats - 1x12, 1x10, 1x8, 1x6, 1x4 reps for each leg

7. Super set exercise 5 and 6 together

8. Exercise 7 - bench press decline - 1x10, 1x8, 1x6, 1x4, 1x2 reps

9. Exercise 8 - incline fly - 1x10, 1x8, 1x6, 1x4, 1x2 reps

10. Super set exercise 8 and 9 together

11. Running on spot fast – 1x30, 1x30, 1x30, 1x30 seconds

12. Exercise 22 - side laterals - 1x10, 1x8, 1x6, 1x4, 1x2 reps

13. Exercise 24 - bent over laterals - 1x10, 1x8, 1x6, 1x4, 1x2 reps

14. Super set exercise 12 and 13

15. Cool down for 5 - 6 minutes

* super-set - doing one set of pullovers then doing one set of one arm rows right after before going back to pullovers

Workout 3 – Level 3

1. Warm- up for 5-6 minutes

2. Exercise 4 - Bent over rows – 1x15, 1x12, 1x10, 1x8, 1x6 reps

3. Exercise 20- Side to side lunge – 1x15, 1x14, 1x13, 1x12 reps

4. Exercise 5 – Flat bench press - 1x15, 1x12, 1x10, 1x8, 1x6 reps

5. Exercise 12- Holding dumbbell squats - 1x15, 1x12, 1x10, 1x8, 1x6 reps

6. Exercise 25- Upright rows - 1x15, 1x12, 1x10, 1x8, 1x6 reps

7. Running on spot – 1 minute x 3

8. Cool down for 5-6 minutes

9. Static stretching

Workout 4 – Level 3

1. Warm up for 5-6 minutes

2. Exercise 11- dumbbell pullovers – 1x20, 1x15, 1x12, 1x10, 1x10 reps

3. Exercise 13 - front squats – 1x20, 1x15, 1x12, 1x10, 1x10 reps

4. Super set exercise 2 and 3 together

5. Push ups – 1x20, 1x20, 1x15, 1x15, 1x10 reps

6. Exercise 18 - stiff legged deadlifts – 1x16, 1x14, 1x12, 1x10, 1x10 reps

- do not do the last set if your low back gets tired from the higher reps

7. Supers set exercise 5 and 6 together

8. Exercise 30 - lying extensions - 1x20, 1x15, 1x12, 1x10, 1x10 reps

9. Jumping jacks – 1x30, 1x30, 1x30, 1x30 reps

10. Exercise 33- hammer curls – 1x20, 1x15, 1x12, 1x10 reps

11. Cool down for 5-6 minutes

12. Static stretching after

DUMBBELL WORKOUTS FOR WOMEN

Women don't sweat, they glow. After training hundreds of women, some don't mind the term sweating while others hate it. Regardless if you hate the term or not, you are going to sweat after doing these workouts. Here are eight workouts for you to do at your home.

Two Beginner Workouts

Workout 1 – Level 1

1. Warm up for 5-6 minutes

2. Exercise 14 - plie squats – 1x15, 1x12, 1x10 reps

3. Exercise 1 - one arm rows -1x15, 1x12, 1x10 reps

4. Jumping jacks – 1x20, 1x20, 1x20 reps

5. Exercise 5 – flat bench presses - 1x15, 1x12, 1x10 reps

6. Exercise 18 - stiff legged dead lifts - 1x15, 1x12, 1x10 reps

7. Jumping jacks - 1x20, 1x20, 1x20 reps

8. Exercise 26 - calf rocks - 1x15, 1x12, 1x10 reps

9. Exercise 25 - upright rows - 1x15, 1x12, 1x10 reps

10. Exercise 29 – one arm kickbacks - 1x15, 1x12, 1x10 reps for each side

11. Exercise 32 - alternate curls - 1x15, 1x12, 1x10 reps

12. Cool down - 5-6 minutes

13. Static stretching after

Workout 2 – Level 1

1. Warm up for 5-6 minutes

2. Exercise 13 - front squats – 1x20, 1x15, 1x12 reps

3. Exercise 2 - deadlifts - 1x16, 1x14, 1x12 reps

4. Running on spot - 1 minute

5. Exercise 8 - Incline fly - 1x20, 1x15, 1x12 reps

6. Exercise 19 – lying leg curls -1x20, 1x15, 1x12 reps

7. Running on spot - 1 minute

8. Exercise 20 - side lunges – 1x10, 1x10, 1x10 reps

9. Exercise 24 - bent over laterals - 1x20, 1x15, 1x12 reps

10. Cool down - 5-6 minutes

11. Static stretching

Two Intermediate Workouts

Workout 1 – Level 2

1. Warm up for 5-6 minutes

2. Exercise 15 - V-up leg extensions – 1x15, 1x12, 1x10, 1x10 reps

3. Exercise 11 - pullovers - 1x15, 1x12, 1x10, 1x10 reps

4. Super set exercise 2 and 3

5. Jumping jacks – 1x30, 1x30, 1x30 reps

6. Exercise 6 – incline bench press - 1x15, 1x12, 1x10, 1x10 reps

7. Exercise 18 - stiff legged dead lifts - 1x15, 1x12, 1x10, 1x10 reps

8. Super set exercise 6 and 7

9. Jumping jacks – 1x30, 1x30, 1x30 reps

10. Exercise 21 - shoulder presses - 1x15, 1x12, 1x10, 1x10 reps

11. Exercise 29 - one arm kickbacks - 1x15, 1x12, 1x10, 1x10 reps

12. Super set exercise 10 and 11

13. Exercise 32 - alternate curls - 1x15, 1x12, 1x10 reps

14. Cool down for 5-6 minutes

15. Static stretching

Workout 2 – level 2

1. Warm up for 5-6 minutes

2. Exercise 12 – holding dumbbell squats – 1x20, 1x15, 1x12, 1x10 reps

3. Exercise 4 – bent over rows - 1x20, 1x15, 1x12, 1x10 reps

4. Super set exercise 2 and 3

5. Running on spot for 1 minute

6. Exercise 9 - flat fly - 1x20, 1x15, 1x12, 1x10 reps

7. Exercise 19 – lying leg curls - 1x20, 1x15, 1x12, 1x10 reps

8. Super set exercise 6 and 7

9. Running on spot 1 minute

10. Exercise 20 - side to side lunges - 1x15, 1x12, 1x10, 1x10 reps

11. Exercise 24 - bent over laterals - 1x20, 1x15, 1x12, 1x10 reps

12. Super set exercise 10 and 11

13. Running on spot 1 minute

14. Cool down for 5-6 minutes

15. Static stretching

Four Advanced Workouts

Workout 1 – Level 3

1. Warm up for 5-6 minutes

2. Exercise 14 - plie squats – 1x15, 1x12, 1x10, 1x8, 1x6 reps

3. Exercise 9 - flat fly - 1x15, 1x12, 1x10, 1x8, 1x6 reps

4. Super set exercise 2 and 3

5. Running on the spot or cardio for 1 minute x 2 times

6. Exercise 18 - stiff legged dead lifts -1x15, 1x12, 1x10, 1x8, 1x6 reps

7. Exercise 1 - one arm rows - 1x15, 1x12, 1x10, 1x8, 1x6 reps

8. Super set exercise 6 and 7

9. Jumping jacks – 1x30, 1x30, 1x30, 1x30 reps

10. Exercise 19 - lying leg curls - 1x15, 1x12, 1x10, 1x8, 1x6 reps

11. Exercise 23 - rotation presses - 1x15, 1x12, 1x10, 1x8, 1x6 reps

12. Super set exercise 10 and 11

13. Running on the spot - 1 minute x 2 times

14. Exercise 31 - bench dips -1x15, 1x12, 1x10, 1x8, 1x6 reps

15. Exercise 34 - one arm curls - 1x14, 1x12, 1x10, 1x8 reps

16. Super set exercise 14 and 15

17. Cool down for 5-6 minutes

18. Static stretching

Workout 2 – level 3

1. Warm up for 5-6 minutes

2. Exercise 15 - v-up leg extensions – 1x20, 1x15, 1x12, 1x10, 1x8 reps

3. Exercise 20 - side to side lunge - 1x15, 1x12, 1x10, 1x8 reps

4. Super set exercise 2 and 3

5. Knee push ups – 1x20, 1x15, 1x12, 1x10, 1x8 reps

6. Exercise 11 - pullovers - 1x20, 1x15, 1x12, 1x10, 1x8 reps

7. Super set exercise 5 and 6

8. Running on the spot – 1 minute x 5 times

9. Exercise 27 - one legged calf raises - 1x20, 1x15, 1x12, 1x10, 1x10 reps for each side

10. Super set exercise 8 and 9

11. Cool down for 5 - 6 minutes

12. Static stretching

Workout 3 – Level 3

1. Warm up for 5-6 minutes

2. Exercise 16 - split squats – 1x14, 1x12, 1x10, 1x8, 1x6 reps for each side

3. Exercise 2 - deadlifts - 1x15, 1x12, 1x10, 1x8, 1x6 reps

4. Jumping jacks – 1x30, 1x10, 1x30, 1x30 reps

5. Exercise 6 - Incline bench press - 1x15, 1x12, 1x10, 1x8, 1x6 reps

6. Exercise 19 - hamstring curls - 1x15, 1x12, 1x10, 1x8, 1x6 reps

7. Jumping jacks – 1x30, 1x30, 1x30, 1x30 reps

8. Exercise 22 – side laterals – 1x15, 1x12, 1x10, 1x8 reps

9. Exercise 26 - calf rocks – 1x15, 1x12, 1x10, 1x10 reps

10. Cool down for 5-6 minutes

11. Static stretching

Workout 4 – Level 3

1. Warm up for 5-6 minutes

2. Exercise 1 - one arm rows – 1x20, 1x15, 1x12, 1x10, 1x8 reps

3. Exercise 13 - front squats – 1x20, 1x15, 1x12, 1x10, 1x8 reps

4. Super set exercise 2 and 3

5. Running on spot fast – 1 minute x 5 times

6. Exercise 10 - decline fly -1x20, 1x15, 1x12, 1x10, 1x8 reps

7. Super set exercise 5 and 6

8. Exercise 25 – upright rows – 1x20, 1x15, 1x12, 1x10 reps

9. Running on spot fast – 1 minute x 5 times

10. Super set exercise 8 and 9

11. Exercise 28 – overhead extensions – 1x20, 1x15, 1x12, 1x10, 1x8 reps

12. Exercise 34 – one arm concentrations curls - 1x18, 1x15, 1x12 reps for each side

13. Cool down for 5-6 minutes

14. Static stretching

TRAINING SCHEDULES

Working out whether it be resistance or cardio training with no direction is like trying to start a business with no business plan. It usually does not end very well. Here are 2 eight week training programs to follow for both men and women.

8 WEEK TRAINING SCHEDULE FOR MEN

Men's Beginner Two Week Schedule To Follow

Week 1

Monday: Workout 1 -Level 1

Tuesday: cardio + core(abs)

Wednesday: Workout 2 – Level 1

Thursday: rest

Friday: Workout 1 -Level 1

Saturday: rest

Sunday: cardio + core(abs)

Week 2

Monday: Workout 1 -Level 1

Tuesday: cardio + core

Wednesday: Workout 2 – Level 1

Thursday: rest

Friday: Workout 1 -Level 1

Saturday: rest

Sunday: cardio + core

Intermediate Two Week Schedule To Follow

Week 3

Monday: Workout 1 - Level 2

Tuesday: cardio + core

Wednesday: Workout 2 -Level 2

Thursday: rest

Friday: Workout 1 - Level 2

Saturday: rest

Sunday: cardio + core

Week 4

Monday: Workout 1 - Level 2

Tuesday: cardio + core

Wednesday: Workout 2 -Level 2

Thursday: rest

Friday: Workout 1 - Level 2

Saturday: rest

Sunday: cardio + core

Advanced Four Week Schedule To Follow

Week 5

Monday: Workout 1- Level 3

Tuesday: cardio + core

Wednesday: Workout 2 – Level 3

Thursday: rest

Friday: Workout 1 – Level 3

Saturday: rest

Sunday: cardio + core

Week 6

Monday: Workout 1- Level 3

Tuesday: cardio + core

Wednesday: Workout 2 – Level 3

Thursday: rest

Friday: Workout 1 – Level 3

Saturday: rest

Sunday: cardio + core

Week 7

Monday: Workout 4- Level 3

Tuesday: cardio + core

Wednesday: Workout 3 – Level 3

Thursday: rest

Friday: Workout 4 – Level 3

Saturday: rest

Sunday: cardio + core

Week 8

Monday: Workout 4- Level 3

Tuesday: cardio + core

Wednesday: Workout 3 – Level 3

Thursday: rest

Friday: Workout 4 – Level 3

Saturday: rest

Sunday: cardio + core

8 WEEK TRAINING SCHEDULE FOR WOMEN

Women's Beginner Two Week Schedule To Follow

Week 1

Sunday: rest

Monday: Workout 1 -Level 1

Tuesday: cardio + core(abs)

Wednesday: Workout 2 - Level 1

Thursday: cardio + core(abs)

Friday: Workout 1 – Level 1

Saturday: rest

Week 2

Sunday: rest

Monday: Workout 1 -Level 1

Tuesday: cardio + core(abs)

Wednesday: Workout 2 - Level 1

Thursday: rest

Friday: Workout 1 – Level 1

Saturday: cardio + core(abs)

Intermediate Two Week Schedule To Follow

Week 3

Sunday: rest

Monday: Workout 1 -Level 2

Tuesday: cardio + core

Wednesday: Workout 2 – Level 2

Thursday: cardio + core

Friday: Workout 1 – level 2

Saturday: rest

Week 4

Sunday: rest

Monday: Workout 1 -Level 2

Tuesday: cardio + core

Wednesday: Workout 2 – Level 2

Thursday: rest

Friday: Workout 1 – level 2

Saturday: cardio + core

Advanced Four Week Schedule To Follow

Week 5

Sun: rest

Mon: Workout 1- Level 3

Tues: cardio + core

Wed: Workout 2 – Level 3

Thurs: cardio + core

Fri: Workout 1- Level 3

Sat: rest

Week 6

Sun: rest

Mon: Workout 1- Level 3

Tues: cardio + core

Wed: Workout 2 – Level 3

Thurs: rest

Fri: Workout 1- Level 3

Sat: cardio + core

Week 7

Sun: rest

Mon: Workout 3- Level 3

Tues: cardio + core

Wed: Workout 4 – Level 3

Thurs: cardio + core

Fri: Workout 3- Level 3

Sat: rest

Week 8

Sun: rest

Mon: Workout 3- Level 3

Tues: cardio + core

Wed: Workout 4 – Level 3

Thurs: rest

Fri: Workout 3- Level 3

Sat: cardio + core

CONCLUSION

After completing the eight week training program, I hope you have gained some muscle, lost some fat, and have greater self confidence. There is no secret to staying in shape. Consistency is the number factor in achieving your goals whether it be weight loss or to gain muscle. You can use a wide variety of equipment but in order for that equipment to be effective, it must be used properly.

The proper equation for results is cardio + resistance training + diet. Once you have achieved the proper balance, nothing is impossible. Remember this equation and you will understand and see how easy it is to maintain a healthy body weight.

ABOUT THE AUTHOR

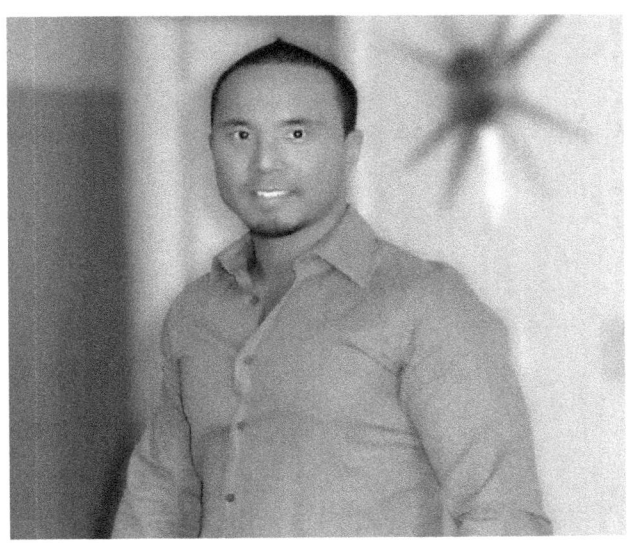

Paul Nam has been in the fitness industry and a personal trainer for over 20 years. He started bodybuilding at the age of 18 and became the Junior Mackenzie Bodybuilding Champion at 19. He has since then competed in over 25 bodybuilding, fitness, and martial arts competitions. He has trained in Olympic style boxing, Brazilian jui-jitsu, muay thai, wrestling, and holds a red belt in tae kwon do.

Paul owns a fitness studio in Toronto, builds mobile training apps, and is now writing a series of books. He is also bringing new fitness products to the world.

CERTIFICATIONS:

Can-Fit Pro -Personal Training Specialist

Children's Fitness Coach

Fascia – Movement And Assessments

YMCA - Fitness Instructor

Yoga - Level 1

Pilates Mat - Level 1

Fitness Kickboxing - Level 1

CPR & First Aid

Nutritionist

Sports Consultant